HERBAL HEALING

A PRACTICAL INTRODUCTION TO MEDICINAL HERBS

HERBAL HEALING

A PRACTICAL INTRODUCTION TO MEDICINAL HERBS

MICHAEL HALLOWELL

FOREWORD BY JACK HO

Avery Publishing Group

Garden City Park, New York

Cover Design: William Gonzalez
Original Illustrations: Graham Fleming

ISBN 0-89529-604-7

First published in Great Britain by Ashgrove Press Limited

Printed in the United States of America

10   9   8

DEDICATED

To my wife Jackie
and to my three sons
Martyn-Daniel
Simon-Peter
and Aaron-James

CONTENTS

ACKNOWLEDGEMENTS

Without the help of the following individuals and organizations, this work could never have been completed. There are others whom I cannot mention, simply because to do so would require a separate volume in itself. To those mentioned here – and all those who are not – my deepest thanks.

The Science Department of the United States Embassy in London, for information regarding health organizations in the United States of America.

The staff of the Public Information Department of the Chinese Embassy in London, for their valuable advice concerning plant medicine research in the Peoples Republic of China, and also for taking the time to furnish me with names and addresses of various Chinese medical academies.

The staff at the Public Information Department of the Russian Embassy in London for information regarding Soviet research into alternative medical therapies.

Ian Hopkins, amateur. historian, for information concerning folk-medicine and scientific interest in herbal medicines in Eastern Europe.

Jack Ho Ph.D, DH, D.Hom., for writing the foreword to this book and reading through the final manuscript.

Graham Fleming and Catherine Wood for preparing the illustrations that accompany the text.

I am also deeply indebted to the following individuals and organizations who kindly supplied me with information regarding their aims and activities.

David Cummings, Secretary of The British Institute of Health
The Faculty of Herbal Medicine
The International College of Natural Health and Sciences
The Health Practitioners Association
The Dominion Herbal College in Canada.

Occasionally, getting information about a particular herb or herbal product proved difficult. The following companies and institutions went to considerable trouble – and at their own expense – to provide me with material that would fill the gaps.

Brewhurst's Health Food Supplies of Rochdale, and Arun Products Ltd., of Bognor Regis for information regarding Slippery Elm (*Ulmus fulva*).
The Institute For Plant Medicines Research.
The Cumbrian Farmers Association for collating botanical and statistical information regarding the different varieties of Onion (*Allium cepa*)

I am also deeply indepted to the following people who, although not directly involved with the writing of this book, were nevertheless a tremendous source of encouragement.

The staff of the Herbal Quarterly magazine, New Fane, Vermont, U.S.A., for taking seriously my thoughts on *Borago officinalis*. Richard Capstick, Editor of Tynesider and Wearsider magazines, for helping me keep my sense of balance during my heady days as a young medical columnist.

And last, but most certainly not least, all my family.

FOREWORD

The subject of herbal or botanic medicine has been debated continually over the millenia, and will, I am sure, continue to be debated as long as the plant life of our globe subsists. One thing is certain; we wouldn't be here to debate anything without it!

For many centuries now, herbal medicines have provided the firm ground of efficiency on which physicians have treated all the ailments that affect the human body. Now, herbal medicine is one of the most effective branches of the 'alternative' medical profession, and it has established itself as a firm competitor against orthodoxy. This is not to say that there should be a bitter rivalry between the orthodox and unorthodox professions; would that they should associate in harmony for the promotion of holistic medicine as a united body!

As a keen herbalist myself, and a devoted student of other alternative therapies, I feel that there is a real need for a basic introduction to the subject. Fortunately, Michael Hallowell had – without my realization – written just such an introductory guide.

If there is one pervading strength to this work, it must surely be the purely logical manner in which it has been compiled. In it, the author elucidates the effects of herbal medicines and why they occur. Then he moves on to show us how those very herbs can be collected, stored and eventually turned into remedies for everyday use. Furthermore, there are sections covering methods of application and dosage, etc., in which every statement is fully explained, and every idea or concept sufficiently covered.

The unique presentation of the material and its fresh format make this book truly different. It will, I am sure, prove to be a pleasurable and instructive introduction to the many people who are just beginning to discover the healing power of plants.

Jack Ho Ph.D, DH, D.Hom.

INTRODUCTION

Herbal or plant medicine has a long and fascinating history. Indeed, it is unlikely that there has ever been a time when – perhaps with the exception of the Garden of Eden – mankind has not utilized plants in his immutable struggle to conquer disease.

We know that the ancient Egyptians were conversant with the properties of such herbs as Cinnamon, Peppermint, Caraway, Aniseed, Terebinth, Lemon Verbena and Cydonia. Various papyrii have been unearthed detailing the use of these and other herbs in the treatment of ulcers, migraine and other ailments.

Sumerian clay tablets have been discovered that list over three hundred plants with medicinal properties. Elderberry, Pomegranate, Lettuce and Fennel were highly valued by contemporary Herbalists, and these plants were carefully scrutinized before purchase to ensure that they were of supernal quality.

The ancient Hebrews too, had an astonishing knowledge of herbal lore and plant-medicine properties. The Bible itself mentions a plethora of medical herbs including Myrrh, Wormwood and Fig, and occasionally gives detailed accounts of their use by physicians. There is, in fact, a considerable amount of internal evidence within the Scriptures to indicate that several herbs not indigenous to Palestine were imported at great cost. Amongst these was the highly-prized *Panax quinquefolia*, or, as it is more commonly called, Ginseng.

A detailed history of herbal medicine would fill many volumes in itself. Suffice it to say that only during the last one hundred and fifty years have we seen traditional medicine finally usurped from its place by the advent of mineral drug therapy.

Only thirty years ago there were those who predicted that herbal medicine was painfully enduring its final death throes. Even some Herbalists themselves had the uneasy feeling that the age of the 'quick cure' would, once and for all time, relegate herbal therapy to

xiv   *Herbal Healing*

the musty pages of some long forgotten book upon the library shelf.

Fortunately, this scenario never became a reality. Disenchanted with the severe side-effects of many modern medicines, people are one again turning to the plant kingdom for natural drugs that work in harmony with the body instead of violently suppressing its natural process and functions. Herbal medicine is currently undergoing a renaissance, and there is no indication that the current trend towards *vis medicatrix naturae* is slowing down.

This book is designed to impart to you some of the knowledge that experienced Herbalists have accumulated down through the centuries, and in an effort to make the volume of interest to everyone, I have included much information that may be new even to those who have a deep understanding of the subject, whilst at the same time compiling the volume in such a way that those who are only just beginning to comprehend the healing power of plants will be able to read the volume from start to finish without becoming 'lost off', so to speak.

Included in the text is a considerable amount of data that will be of interest to students of botany, plant pharmacology and pharmacognosy. However, there has also been included a great deal of herbal lore which will be interesting to those who are intrigued by the sociological aspects of 'folk-medicine'.

Many ethnic groups such as the Basques, Bedouins and Romanies have, albeit by necessity, developed the practice of plant medicine to a high degree. Although traditional 'folk-healers' do not often demonstrate any great knowledge of anatomy, physiology or any other specific medical discipline, it must be said that their cures have in times past produced some spectacular results, and still do today.

One of the most interesting characteristics of herbal medicine is that the herbs used by each practitioner are decided upon largely by his geographical location rather than his personal choice. Herbalists in the U.S.A. for instance, use many plant medicines that are unavailable here in the United Kingdom, and of which I have only a superficial knowledge. The same principle also applies in reverse. I stock many herbs that cannot be found in the U.S.A. simply because the climate does not engender their growth.

Because of the above facts, it will be self-evident that many of the reported uses recorded within the general text of this book are made not on the basis of my own personal experience but on that of my colleagues in other countries. Where this is the case, I have been careful only to glean my information from the most reputable sources. Indeed, it is these differences in *materia medica* that ensures that research into plant medicines does not become stagnant, but rather remains refreshingly diversified.

In conclusion I will say this: when my first published piece on the subject of herbal medicine appeared in print some years ago, I committed myself 'to the wholehearted belief that within the plant kingdom lie safer, cheaper and far more beneficial alternatives to our pernicious orthodox drugs.' Since that time, I have neither seen nor heard anything that has caused me to change my mind.

In this book we will examine more closely just such alternatives. I hope that you will find it at least entertaining, and hopefully of some practical benefit.

MICHAEL J. HALLOWELL
West Boldon, Tyne and Wear

Part One

A WORD OF CAUTION

One of the greatest advantages of herbal medicine as a therapy is that it is – when administered correctly – completely safe. Unfortunately, some amateur herbalists have, in their sincere desire to publicize the beneficial qualities of plant medicines, fostered the totally erroneous idea that herbal medicines can be swallowed in a spirit of cavalier abandon without causing the slightest harm. This notion is both incorrect and dangerous.

Despite the fact that herbal preparations are far safer in general than orthodox medicines, they must still be used with discrimination. Some plants are extremely toxic and can cause serious poisoning or even death.

The safety of herbs will be dealt with in more detail in a further chapter, but it is important at this point to lay down several 'golden rules' for the serious student of Herbalism.

1 Unless you are medically qualified to do so, never treat anything but minor ailments at home. Always seek professional advice for serious conditions.

2 Even minor ailments that fail to respond to home treatment should be given the benefit of expert advice.

3 ALWAYS check the dosage of a home-made herbal preparation before you take it. Only take large doses under medical supervision.

4 Never use ANY herb for medicinal purposes unles you have identified it correctly and are sure it is safe.

5 Finally, remember this golden rule of self-medication: IF IN DOUBT, DON'T!

1 Medicinal Plants And Their Active Constituents

Unlike his modern counterpart, the herbalist of old was not concerned with the complexities of botany or the intricate details of medical science. His success rested largely on two factors; firstly, it was necessary for him to have an accurate knowledge of which herbs cured any given disease, and secondly, he was required to know the exact dose in which the prescribed herb should be administered.

To a large extent the same two principles still form the basis of herbal medicine today, but important advances have been made in recent years which enable those who practise the art of plant medicine to gain a greater understanding of the herbs that they use. Theophrastus, Celsus and more recently John Gerard and Nicholas Culpeper, were all expert herbalists who undoubtedly had a detailed understanding of the effects of plant medicines on the human frame, but we today have the added advantage of knowing not just what those physiological effects are, but also why they occur.

There is no mystique about the therapeutic value of plants. Their actions within the body are governed by sound scientific principles. To establish exactly why herbal drugs work we must first take a look at their chemical constituents.

Concerning matters medical it is convenient to divide the plant kingdom into three groups: the Acute Toxic, the Inert, and the Therapeutic.

ACUTELY TOXIC PLANTS

Generally speaking, these plants have very little in the way of medicinal virtues, and those that do normally have their therapeutic properties overshadowed by the fact that they are extremely toxic even when taken in small amounts.

Examples of this type are some of the three hundred species of Lupin, the two species of the Laburnum tree (*L. alpinum* and *L. anagyroides*), and *Strychnos toxifera* (Curare Poison Nut).

INERT PLANTS

These are plants that, although affecting the human physiology as all ingested substances must inevitably do, do not produce any immediately observable effects (either therapeutic or toxic), even when taken in quite large amounts.

Most foodstuffs of an organic or vegetable nature fall into this category. Examples are the Potato (*Solanum tuberosum*) and the Cabbage (*Brassica oleracea*).

THERAPEUTIC PLANTS

The third grouping, and the one that specifically concerns us, is that of the therapeutic plants. These are herbs that have decidedly medicinal values that can be utilised in the treatment of disease.

The line between inert plants and those that are classed as therapeutic is notoriously difficult to draw, perhaps impossible. For example, Garlic (*Allium sativum*) is universally accepted as both a medicinal herb and a culinary one, whilst its close relative the Onion (*Allium cepa*) is normally regarded only as a vegetable. In recent years scientific research has discovered that the Onion too has therapeutic virtues. In time, that plant may gain its rightful place in both groups just as Garlic has done.

It is also difficult to differentiate between Therapeutic plants and Toxic ones. Some herbs that are decidedly therapeutic in their action may also be toxic when taken in excess.

Of course, what constitutes a toxic dose of a normally therapeutic herb depends largely on the herb in question. Sometimes, the toxic dose may be two or three hundred times the medicinal dosage, and thus it may be possible, although I certainly do not recommend it, to swallow large amounts of the plant and not suffer any immediate symptoms of toxicity.

Conversely, some herbs have a toxic dose so close to the therapeutic one that any attempt by the layman at self-medication will be likely to end in disaster.

Although most species can easily be identified as belonging to one of the three categories (or occasionally two), some must be classified purely on the personal opinion of the reader.

Experienced herbalists are aware that when two herbs or more are prescribed together, their individual properties react together in such a way that other effects are produced that are not normally found when either of the herbs are prescribed separately. This chemical reaction is sometimes called synergism, or as a Canadian herbalist once put it, 'two plus two makes five'.

PLANT CHEMICALS AND THEIR EFFECTS

No two plants have the same effect upon the body by virtue of the fact that the chemical make-up of every single species is different. If we are to understand how herbs can produce such a variety of effects then we must, as previously stated, examine the chemicals that they contain.

The Alkaloids

Characteristics: Alkaloids are a chemically stable group of organic substances that

CONTAIN NITROGEN   ARE SENSITIVE TO HEAT   ARE CRYS-
TALLINE IN STRUCTURE   ARE TASTELESS AND ODOURLESS

There are a large number of alkaloids – several hundred actually – and others are being discovered on an almost daily basis. They have a very complicated chemical structure and the majority of them are extremely toxic.

EXAMPLE: *Atropa belladonna* (Deadly Nightshade).
CONTAINS: The alkaloid *Atropine*.
USES: Great use has been made of this substance as an antispasmodic, and its use by both orthodox physi-

cians and Herbalists alike in the treatment of diseases
of the nervous system is well known.

EXAMPLE: *Papaver somniferum* (Poppy).
CONTAINS: The alkaloids *Morphine, Thebaine, Codeine, Rebaine,
Narcotine* and *Papaverine*.
USES: Used for relieving muscular spasms, controlling
irritating coughs and as pain-killers.

Curiously, no satisfactory explanation has ever been advanced as
to why alkaloids are present in plant material in the first place. They
undoubtedly have an important function, but it has yet to be
discovered.

The Vitamins

Characteristics: All medicinal herbs possess a quota of vitamins, and
these too influence the effect of the plant upon the human
physiology. Some herbs contain large amounts of one particular
vitamin. Comfrey contains the B complex in generous amounts, and
the dandelion contains a massive 13,650 International Units of
Vitamin A and 40mg. of Vitamin C per 100g.

The therapeutic effects of vitamins are well documented, and any
ailment caused by their deficiency can normally be rectified by
prescribing a herb that is rich in the required substance.

VITAMIN A Chemical name carotene. Fat soluble.
Required daily amount: U.K. 2,500 I.U.s; U.S.A.
5,000 I.U.s.
Health-promoting qualities: good eyesight, healthy
digestive system and respiratory organs, good skin
texture.
Deficiency causes: scaling of the skin, burning
sensation in the eyes, susceptibility to infection.

Good herbal or plant sources: Dandelion greens,
other leafy green vegetables.

VITAMIN B1   Chemical name thiamine. Water soluble.
Required daily amount: U.K. 1.4mg; U.S.A. 1.5mg.
Health promoting qualities: converts starch to energy, keeps nervous system healthy.
Deficiency causes: poor digestion, headaches, tongue discoloration, constipation.

Good herbal or plant sources: Comfrey and Borage. Comfrey (*Symphytum officinale*) contains 0.5mg per 100g; and Borage (*Borago officinalis*) 0.4mg. More accessible sources are wholegrain cereals, nuts, peas and oranges.

VITAMIN B2   Chemical name riboflavin. Water soluble.
Required daily amount; U.K. 1.7mg; U.S.A. 1.7mg.
Health-promoting qualities: necessary to maintain healthy eyes, skin and nervous system.
Deficiency causes: muscular tremors, vertigo, tongue inflammation.

Good herbal or plant sources: Spinach 20mg per 100mg; Borage 3mg; Texas Snake Root (*Aristolochia serpentaria*) 18mg.

VITAMIN B3   Chemical name niacin. Water soluble.
Required daily amount: U.K. 18mg; U.S.A. 20mg.
Health-promoting qualities: increases brain efficiency and keeps nerve tissue in good condition.
Deficiency causes: mental disorientation, tongue discolouration, vomiting, halitosis and constipation.

Good herbal or plant sources: Indian Corn (*Zea mays*) 12mg; Dandelion greens 18mg per 100g.

VITAMIN B6   Chemical name pyridoxine. Water soluble.
Required daily amount: U.K. none; U.S.A. 2mcg.
Health-promoting qualities: helps body assimilate

protein material, keeps the skin, muscle tissue and nervous system healthy.
Deficiency causes: skin sores, headaches, anaemia.

Good herbal or plant sources: Corn Oil and Cabbage, and also Comfrey and Polypody Root (Polydium vulgare).

VITAMIN B12   Chemical name cyanocobalamin. Water soluble.
Required daily amount: U.K. none; U.S.A. 6mcg.
Health promoting qualities: helps body to absorb proteins, carbohydrates, minerals and fats. Also aids memory function and the process of cell renewal.
Deficiency causes: pernicious anaemia, loss of memory, vomiting, tingling sensations in the extremities and symptoms of Parkinsonism.

Good herbal or plant sources: virtually none. Most B12 is found in meat or dairy products, and a little is manufactured by 'friendly bacteria' in the large intestine. There is one noticeable exception to this. Comfrey contains 0.7mg of B12 per 100g.

VITAMIN C   Chemical name ascorbic acid. Water soluble.
Required daily amount: U.K. 30mg; U.S.A. 60mg.
Health promoting qualities: helps build new connective tissue, strengthens the blood vessels, keeps skin and muscles healthy.
Deficiency causes: scurvy and easy bruising of the skin, prolonged healing of broken bones, tiredness and impaired resistance to infection.

Good herbal or plant sources: Dandelion greens or roots, Parsley (*Alchemilla arvensis*) 150mg per 100g; and Sorrel (*Rumex acetosa*).

VITAMIN D   Chemical name cholecalciferol. Fat soluble.
Required daily amount: U.K. 100 I.U.s; U.S.A. 400 U.S.P.s (United States Pharmacopoea Units).

Health promoting qualities: Aids the absorption of calcium and potassium into the bones, prevents the onset of several bone diseases such as osteomalacea, rickets, osteoporosis and Pott's disease.
Deficiency causes: the above mentioned diseases, insomnia, muscle cramps, nose bleeds and dental caries.

Good herbal or plant sources: neglible except for some yeasts and fungi. Fish and eggs are good dietary sources.

VITAMIN E   Chemical name alpha tocopherol. Fat soluble.
Required daily amounts: U.K. none; U.S.A. 30 I.U.s.
Health promoting qualities: protects certain nutrients such as polyunsaturated fats from destruction before the body has been able to digest them, strengthens blood vessel walls and increases the efficiency with which the blood is oxygenated.
Deficiency causes: sporadic (although normally minor) internal bleeding.

Good herbal or plant sources: Corn Oil, Barley, Rye, Lettuce, various nuts and beans. E can also be found in Chamomile (*Anthemis nobilis* and *Chamomilla matricaria*) and Sesame (*Sesamum indicum*).

The Bitter Principles

Characteristics: 'Bitters' are a group of organic chemicals that, although perhaps chemically unrelated, are characterized by being

extremely bitter (although not always unpleasant) to taste
rarely poisonous
anitrogenous

Bitter principles are found throughout the entire plant kingdom, but the two families utilized in a medicinal sense most of all for their bitter substances are

the compositae
the gentianaceae

EXAMPLE: *Strychnos nux-vomica.* (Nux Vomica).
CONTAINS: A variety of bitter principles.
USES: Used as an appetite stimulant to encourage the flow of
              gastric juices, and as a stomachic and nervine. The
              elderly, invalids and the chronically sick often find the
              restorative powers of bitter principles particularly
              beneficial.

IMPORTANT NOTE: Although bitter principles are almost
never poisonous in themselves, this is NOT to say that a plant can be
regarded as non-toxic simply because it tastes bitter, and the example
above illustrates this very clearly. Nux vomica, sometimes called the
Koochla tree, is extremely poisonous and is usually given in only
homoeopathic dosages.

Essential Oils.

Characteristics: Essential or volatile oils are actually waste products
found within the glandular cells of certain plants. Several families
contain an abundance of essential oils. They are

Umbellifereae   Sabiateae
Pinnaceae   Myrtaceae
Tutaceae   Compositae

Some families such as the *Equisetaceae* are almost devoid of
essential essences.

EXAMPLE: *Pimpinella anisum* (Anise Seed).
CONTAINS: ' Oil of Anise Seed.
USES: Used to treat liver and bowel disorders.

The use of volatile oils in the treatment of disease is a highly
specialized medical science. Although some essential oils can be
taken internally, the usual mode of application is to apply the oil to
the skin in a massage rub. The oil is quickly absorbed and acts on the
nervous system. However, essences should never be applied directly
to an open wound as they may cause severe irritation.

Herbal Healing

Minerals.

Characteristics: Minerals are inorganic chemicals absorbed by plants from the ground through their root system. The mineral content of a plant is dependent on a variety of factors including geographical location, temperature, soil conditions, rainfall, proximity to industrial developments and so on.

In relation to the human body the two minerals that concern us most are

Potassium
Calcium

Potassium: The uses of this mineral in the body are manifold. It is necessary for the control of fluid passage in and out of the cell membrane; it aids the smooth contraction of muscular tissue; it prevents an excess of sodium building up in the body; it increases the efficiency with which the liver breaks down fats into fatty acids and glycerol, and also maintains the processes by which glucose is broken down and stored in the liver as glycogen.

EXAMPLE: *Lycopersicon esculentum* (Tomato).
CONTAINS: 360mg of potassium per 100g.
USES: In the treatment of liver diseases and lymph gland disorders.

EXAMPLE: *Asparagus officinalis* (Asparagus).
CONTAINS: 130mg of potassium per 100g.
USES: In the treatment of urinary disorders.

It should be noted here that although the tomato is an excellent source of potassium, THE LEAVES OF THE TOMATO PLANT SHOULD NEVER BE EATEN. They contain an alkaloidal glycoside called solanine which is extremely toxic and CANNOT be destroyed by cooking. Other good vegetable sources of potassium are

Spinaceae oleracea (Spinach) 470mg.
Brasica oleracea (Cabbage) 140mg.
Panax quinquefolia (Ginseng) varies.
Symphytum peregrinum (Russian Comfrey) varies.

Calcium: Calcium is a largely insoluble mineral that is vital to the body in several respects. It is necessary for the formation of bones and teeth, helps build healthy muscle tissue (particularly around the heart) and is instrumental in the blood-clotting process.

The results of calcium deficiency are predictable. Bones become weak and susceptible to fractures, the blood's ability to clot is impaired and cuts tend to bleed lengthily before healing. Also, the circulation of blood to the peripheral organs is reduced and the heart is easily distressed.

EXAMPLE: The three main genera of Sea Kelp, *Macrocystis*, *Laminaria* and *Nereocystis*.

CONTAINS: 1,100mg per 100g.

USES: Treatment of muscular cramps.

Other good sources are *Taraxacum officinalis* (Dandelion) 190 mg per 100g; *Vitis vinifera* (Grape) 100mg; and *Ficus carica* (Fig) 60mg.

Most other trace elements and minerals necessary for our physical well-being can also be found in abundance in the plant kingdom, and although it is not appropriate to discuss them here in any detail, here is a quick resumé.

Fluorine: Necessary in small amounts for the maintainance of healthy bones and teeth. Only traces of this mineral are found in vegetable matter, and although a carefully engineered diet can provide a certain amount, dairy produce and offal are the most accessible sources.

Copper: Without this element, iron cannot be assimilated properly in the body, and thus a copper deficiency can cause anaemia even when the level of iron in the body is adequate. Copper also helps the formation of red blood cells (erythrocytes).

There is an increasing amount of evidence that the presence of copper may produce an increased resistance to certain forms of cancer in the tissues. Those who are deficient in copper show a slightly increased tendency to develop certain types of malignancy, whilst some cancer sufferers who increase their copper intake may have the growth of their cancer slowed down. (It must be noted here that no attempt to artificially raise the level of copper in the body should be made. Copper toxicity is a serious condition that can, amongst other things, cause damage to a developing foetus. Research in the U.K. has established a definite link between copper toxicity and the incidence of spina bifida in the newly born.)

Nevertheless, the possibility that copper may possess anticarcinogenic properties is an interesting one. The herb Comfrey (*Symphytum officinale*) contains significant traces of copper, and has long been pointed at as a herbal 'cancer treatment'. (The British Medical Journal, although not espousing Comfrey as a cancer treatment, did pay homage to its curative properties as far back as 1912. In its June 8th issue it detailed the successful application of Comfrey to a patient with chronic leg ulcers.)

Chlorine: This is a detoxifying element that is necessary for joint mobility. Celery (*Apium graveolens*) is a good source of chlorine, and celery seeds are a popular herbal diuretic and have long been used to flush toxic substances and waste matter from the body.

Silicon: Essential for the development of healthy hair and the prevention of nervous disorders. Lettuce (*Lactuca sativa*) contains substantial amounts of silicon and also the sedative laudanum. Together these make a justifiable reason for giving lettuce tea – an old folk-remedy – to those suffering from hysteria.

Iron: This mineral is essential for the building of the red blood cells and for oxygen assimilation. A deficiency results in anaemia. Many herbs have proved to be a rich source of iron, including *Rubus fruticosus* (Blackberry) 10mg; and the aforementioned Kelp.

Other essential trace elements such as sodium, sulphur, phosphorous and manganese are also found in varying degrees throughout the Plant Kingdom.

Tannins

Characteristics: Tannins are organic by-products of plant growth. They are both

> astringent and
> irritant

Tannins can be found in all the plant families, but mostly the

> Geraniaceae
> Papilionaceae
> Rosaceae

EXAMPLE: *Quercus robur* (Acorn).
CONTAINS: High content, varies from species to species.
USES: Treatment of varicose veins.

Tannins have a variety of medicinal properties. They are used because of their astringent action in the treatment of burns and varicose ulcers, thus giving some credibility to the old folk-remedy that suggests dipping burnt fingers in cold tea which is rich in tannins.

Mucilagens

Characteristics: Mucilagens are by-products of metabolic processes that occur within the plant. They

swell when in contact with water
take on a viscous or plastic constituency

EXAMPLE: *Cetaria islandica* (Iceland Moss).
CONTAINS: High level of mucilagens and two other water-absorbing substances.
USES: Excellent drawing poultice for suppurations.

Chemically speaking, mucilagens are made from long chains of bonded sugars known as polysaccarides. When they are applied to ther skin they act as an emollient, soothing and softening inflamed tissue. Some, such as *Ulmus fulva* (Slippery Elm), are sued to treat intestinal disorders in young children and the eldery or chronically sick.

Saponins

Characteristics: Saponins are naturally occurring plant compounds that are

similar in chemistry to the glycosides
lather-producing when irritated under water

EXAMPLE: *Paris quadrifolia* (Herb Paris).
CONTAINS: Up to 2% of saponins.
USES: Antiseptic.

Many saponins are extremely poisonous and will rapidly cause haemolysis (breaking down of red blood corpuscles) in the circulatory system. However, many common vegetables contain small amounts of saponins, but as they are poorly absorbed by the human digestive system they can be eaten with impunity. Others produce rapid symptoms of toxicity. Herb Paris (see above) is one example, and herbs known to contain saponins should NEVER be eaten until their safety has been fully established.

Glycosides

Characteristics: Glycosides are a complex group of chemicals which contain in their chemical bonding

one non-sugar part (Aglycyn)
one or more sugar parts

There are several types of glycoside, the most common of which are

Digitalis glycosides
Anthraquinone glycosides
Salicylic glycosides
Thiocyanate glycosides
Flavonoid glycosides
Phenolic glycosides

EXAMPLE: *Digitalis purpurea* (Foxglove).
CONTAINS: Cardio-active glycosides.
USES: In the treatment of various heart complaints.

EXAMPLE: *Rheum officinale* (Rhubarb).
CONTAINS: Anthraquinone glycosides.
USES: Anthraquinone glycosides act as laxatives, in the treatment of some bowel disorders.

EXAMPLE: *Viola odorata* (Sweet Violet).
CONTAINS: Salicylic glycosides.
USES: Excellent pain-killers.

EXAMPLE: *Theritata feris* (Blacken Mustard).
CONTAINS: Thiocyanate glycosides.
USES: Used in the treatment of poor circulation.

EXAMPLE: *Sempheris officinale* (African Bells).
CONTAINS: Flavonoid glycosides.
USES: Used to prevent internal bleeding.

EXAMPLE: *Arctostaphylos uva-urse* (Bearberry).
CONTAINS: Phenolic glycosides.
USES: Used to reduce fever, control muscular spasms and increase frequency of urination.

Most glycosides have a powerful action on the heart. The Department of Health does NOT recommend that heart disease is subjected to self-medication, and herbs rich in glycosides must be used with great discretion.

2 The Collection, Preparation and Storage of Medicinal Plants

In recent years there has been a tremendous surge of interest in herbal or botanic medicine, and in consequence a wide variety of ready prepared natural remedies have found their way onto the shelves of herb suppliers, health-food stores and even some chemists. This is something to be commended for obvious reasons, but I think that there is an inherent problem in the commercialization of herbal medicines. We are, in fact, in danger of losing the ability to prepare such medicines on what could well be described as a 'cottage level'.

I have heard it suggested by some herbalists (their title, not mine!) that we should follow the lead of the allopathic profession and simply prescribe herbal medicines that have been produced and neatly packaged by herbal pharmaceutical manufacturers. This would, they say, do away with the unjust image of a Merlin-type figure mixing up some weird and wonderful concoction in a large cauldron whilst bats are flying overhead. I sympathise with this view, and it *is* rather annoying when people keep ringing you at two o'clock in the morning asking you if you can turn their wife into a toad: but I cannot agree that the answer lies in abandoning our ability to prepare individually tailored remedies.

Firstly, we must remember that each patient is a unique individual. No disease follows exactly the same course in one person as it does in another. Thus, each individual reacts differently to any given disease, and it is difficult to believe that one patent medicine can cover all the subtle differences and still be totally effective. Just as the patient should be viewed as unique, so also should the medicine be viewed.

Whilst over-the-counter (O.T.C.) remedies are effective in the treatment of many minor ailments, no herbalist can provide an optimum service to his patients without having the ability to 'tailor make' medicines to suit individual requirements.

Secondly, the ability to make up medicines forms an integral part of the traditional art/science of herbalism. Even if it is retained for no other reason than to educate students of botanic medicine with the ancient skills of their professional ancestors, the ability to create medicines in-house with the simplest equipment will always be a necessity.

COLLECTING MEDICINAL PLANTS

No matter where you live in the world, you will be always be able to find plants that can be cultivated for their medicinal values. Of course, exactly what plants are available in your own locale depends largely on your geographical location. In the North East of England where I live, one can find an almost endless variety of useful herbs, 'weeds' (I detest that word), and shrubs. Even in quite heavily populated towns it is normally possible to find an inexhaustible supply of Dandelion, Groundsel, Chickweed, Coltsfoot, Dock, Plantain and Bindweed.

When collecting plants, especially those that are to be used for medicinal purposes, there are several golden rules to follow. Stick to them, and you can be sure that the plants that you pick will be of the finest quality.

RULE 1   *Identify the plant that you require correctly*
Some herbs are almost indistinguishable from others that have totally different properties. Rosebay Willow-herb (*Chamaenerion angustifolium*) may, to the untrained eye, look suspiciously like Purple Loosestrife (*Lythrum salicaria*), and two members of the Figwort family *Scrophulariaceae* – Yellow Lute *(Odontites lutea)* and Common Cow-wheat (*Melampyrum pratense*) – may also be easily confused by someone who is gingerly taking their first herb-hunting expedition in the fields.

Always take several illustrated pocket-books with you when you are looking for herbs that you are not overly familiar with.

RULE 2   *Never pick herbs within one mile of a public highway*
Some plants such as the Raspberry, Blackberry, Lesser Plantain,

Ground Ivy and Self-Heal have a curious affinity for the lead thrown out by car exhaust fumes. Plants picked by a busy roadside may contain up to two hundred times their natural level of lead.

RULE 3   *Always pick your plants from the correct area*
It is not by coincidence that we may find a field covered with a golden carpet of Coltsfoot or a meadow dotted profusely with clumps of Plantain. If a herb is found to be growing prolifically in a particular area, then we can be sure that the soil in that region is ideally suited for the plant to grow in, and rich in minerals and organic acids or alkalines which promote vigorous and healthy growth.
Always try to pick your herbs from areas such as these.

RULE 4   *Choose carefully the time at which you pick your herbs*
It is a little-known fact that just as the moon's gravitational pull affects the rise and fall of the oceans, it also affects the rise and fall of the sap within the plant. A herb picked at high-tide when the moon is waxing will contain considerably more sap than one picked when the moon is on the wane. Also, herbs that have a naturally high sap content should be picked in the Spring when the plant's water content will be highest.
Time of day is also an important factor. By mid-morning most of the dew has evaporated from the foliage, and this is the best time to pick the plants that you require. Dew-laden herbs tend to develop mould soon after picking.

SELECTING AND PICKING YOUR PLANT

Once you have found the herb that you require growing in a suitable area, it is most important that you select only the best specimens and also that you defoliate the plant in the correct manner. Avoid plants that show any signs of damage or disease. Black spots on the leaves, discoloration of the stem or droopy foliage are some of the tell-tale signs that all is not well.
Unless you require the root of the plant, it is rarely necessary to destroy the whole herb. The Chinese herbalists have an old custom

of only picking the 'dragon's ears' or top two leaves on the plant, and Polish herbalists will always 'leave some for God'; that is, they will never remove the entire plant from the soil, but leave the rootstock at least to flourish again. Both ideas are to be encouraged because they promote vigorous growth and ensure that the species population does not become depleted.

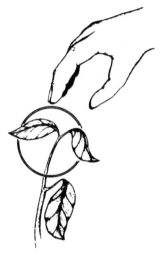

Only picking new growth ensures that the whole plant is not destroyed.

When removing the foliage, only choose tender young leaves that have a healthy appearance. Old leaves tend to be tough and battle-scarred due to exposure to harsh winters. Leaves from biennial plants should, when possible, be picked in their second year.

Flowerheads are particularly prone to damage, especially from marauding insects. The best time to pick flowerheads is in the early morning, but be sure to dry them at the soonest opportunity to prevent moulding taking place. Avoid blooms that are starting to lose their petals as they are past their best.

Removing bark is perhaps the most delicate operation, because if it is removed in the wrong manner the entire plant may die. In the Autumn – the best time to remove bark — carefully select the tree or shrub that you require. Then, with a sharp blade or small hack-saw carefully remove smaller branches from the top and outer areas of the plant. Bark is much more easily stripped from new stemmage and branches.

Do not attempt to remove bark from the branches whilst they are still attached to the tree. You may accidentally 'run' the strip of bark down the trunk and leave the tree open to infection from parasites, fungi or disease.

Once you have removed the parts of the plant that you require – that is the leaves, stem, root, bark, seeds or flowerhead – store them in small cotton or muslin bags for transportation. NEVER mix two or more herbs in the same bag. You would be amazed how two herbs that looked entirely different in the field can look confusingly similar on the kitchen bench!

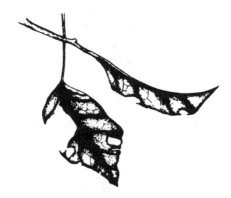

Diseased and pest-ridden leaves like these should be avoided at all costs.

Be careful not to crush or damage the leaves during transportation. A wire frame placed inside the collecting bag can help prevent this.

DRYING AND PRESERVING

Having collected your herbs, it is important that you prepare them for storage as soon as possible. Every home herbalist has his or her own techniques and favourite methods of storing his herbs, and some of them are quite simple. For instance, you can simply add the fresh, chopped herb to some white vinegar, and within a week or two you will have an aromatic condiment that will not only taste good but will also contain all the goodness of the herb that you added to it.

However, by far the most popular means of preserving herbs is by drying. By removing the moisture from the cellular structure of the plant you trap the 'active principles' or therapeutically useful chemicals inside. Also, the plant is impervious to mould, disease and other problems. Dried herbs can – depending on the species – be stored for anything up to five years without a loss of potency taking place.

Basically, there are two methods of drying, both of which have certain advantages and disadvantages. The quicker – and more common – method is indoor oven-drying. The other method, which some herbalists say is preferable, is outdoor frame-drying.

Oven Drying: The main advantage of oven drying is the way in which it saves time. Herbs that would normally take up to six weeks to dry naturally can be dried within an hour indoors.

The herbs should be placed neatly, side by side, on a clean, dry oven tray. A piece of aluminium foil should then be placed over the tray with the reflective side facing innermost. The foil should then be nipped to the edges of the tray, with a small gap being left to allow moisture to escape.

Place the tray into the oven which should be set to a low temperature such as Gas Mk. 2. Every fifteen minutes, remove the tray and turn the herbs over to ensure that the moisture is drawn out evenly from all sides of the plant. If moisture is drawn out through one side more rapidly than the other, burning may occur. Plants should NOT be allowed to burn to a dark brown or black colour. When this happens the potency is detroyed completely and the plant is useless.

The disadvantages of oven-drying are two-fold. Firstly, it is extremely easy to over-dry or burn the herbage. Remember, you are trying to *dry* the herb, not *cook* it. When the leaves or petals crumble gently in your hand without powdering and some or all of the original colour is intact, then the plant is dried sufficiently.

The second disadvantage of oven-drying is that, for various reasons, the herbs lose between ⅓ to ½ of their original potency, compared to their outdoor dried-equivalents which only lose around ¼. When you store an oven-dried herb remember to mark the container in some way so that you are aware of the reduced potency.

Frame Drying: Although this method is more laborious and time-consuming than oven drying, it is often preferred by many experienced herbalist as the loss of potency is somewhat less.

For frame-drying you will need a small wooden or metal box about 3ft square with a glass lid. The base of the frame should be lined with aluminium foil, and there should also be a small, sheltered hole for ventilation. Herbs selected for drying should be placed on the aluminium foil and the lid closed. The plants should be turned once a day until dry.

The frame should, of course, be situated in an area that receives a reasonable amount of sunlight. It should also be absolutely watertight, and all herbs placed in it for drying should be dried gently with a cloth first. *One damp herb placed in the frame may be sufficient to turn the entire batch mouldy.*

Frame drying may take anything between three to six weeks to accomplish.

STORING YOUR HERBS

Having successfully dried your selected herbs, you must now consider by which method you wish to store them, and this is largely determined by the eventual form in which the herb is to be administered. Ointments, for instance, are normally made from finely powdered herbs, whilst tinctures are usually made by submerging the whole root or leaves in alcohol. As a rough guide, I would suggest that the leaves, bark and stem are best comminuted (ground), whilst roots, petals and seeds are best stored whole.

Always ensure that your herbs are thoroughly dried before storage.

Comminution: In herbal parlance, comminution is simply grinding down or powdering of crude herb material. This can be done by the traditional method of using a mortar and pestle or by using an electric grinder.

The mortar and pestle method, although slower, enables the herbalist to determine the eventual fineness of the powder with a great deal more accuracy, but when comminuting herbs for use in ointments or salves it is better to use an electric grinder. This enables the herbalist to achieve a greater degree of fineness and uniformity with the powder.

Storage: This is probably the most important part of the whole procedure. Failure to store your herbs correctly means that all the time and effort spent collecting and drying has been wasted.

Choose the room in which you are to store your herbs extremely carefully. It should be neither damp, cold nor draughty. Do not store your herbs in or near a kitchen, as cooking odours have been known to permeate the most 'impermeable' of containers! I learnt my lesson the hard way during my days as a student herbalist. I once opened a 'sealed' container of Lemon Verbena which normally has an extremely pleasant aroma, only to be greeted by the smell of stale cooking oil. That afternoon my herbs were moved to a cupboard away from the kitchen.

It also goes without saying that dried herbs should NEVER be stored within reach of young children. Remember, they are potential medicines.

Your choice of container is equally important. Some types are totally unsuitable for the storage of dried herbs. Metal containers tend to impart a bitter, metallic flavour and odour to the plants and should never be used. Likewise, clear glass jars allow sunlight to filter through, and prolonged exposure to sunlight will inevitably lead to a loss of potency. Wooden containers can be used occasionally, but these are also prone to absorbing moisture.

Suitable containers can be ceramic, earthenware, brown glass or plastic. Whichever type you use, make sure that they are a) intact and b) airtight. (Some herbalists find that a small amount of powdered chalk wrapped in tissue paper and placed in the container aids against dampness.)

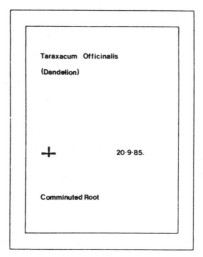

Clear labelling of all storage jars is vitally important.

Labelling: Failure to label storage jars correctly has been the downfall of many a would-be herbalist, because the consequences can, bluntly speaking, be fatal. Every container should display a firmly secured label bearing the following information:

The Date: After several years of storage the potency of dried herbs may deteriorate severely. Make sure that you know the date on which the herbs were picked and dried. This will enable you to determine when your stock needs renewing.

The Name: Always write the Latin, botanical name of the herb on the label. Write the common name also for quick reference, but remember that these 'nicknames' can be confusing. (See *Naming and Identifying Medicinal Plants*).

The Method of Drying: As this effects the potency of the herb, it is vital that you contain this information on your label. A small sign such as + may be used to denote those herbs which have been oven dried, while a sign such as O can be used to identify frame dried herbs.

The Part of the Herb: Always note the part of the herb that you have stored. Comminuted roots, bark and leaves can all look much the same, and as the various parts of a plant can have different medicinal virtues, it is important that you know which is which.

3 Making Herbal Medicines

In the plant kingdom every species is, when found within its natural environment, in a perfect state of chemical balance. Indeed, if this balance – this symbiotic relationship with the external environment – did not exist, the plant could not survive. Unfortunately, this chemical balance is extremely delicate, and if the natural constituency of the plant is disturbed in any way that balance is destroyed.

Of course, the difficulty lies in administering a medicinal herb to a patient *without* destroying that precious balance. Defoliation, drying, heating, exposure to sunlight over a prolonged period after picking, and a host of other processes normally initiate the very thing that should be avoided at all costs – namely, a loss of potency. Logic tells us then, that if a change in the plant's physiology or environment causes a loss of potency, the administration of the herb in it's natural state (i.e. raw) must likewise ensure a *maximum* potency. It is for this reason that herbs should, technically speaking, be eaten raw in the same manner as a vegetable.

Of course, this idea is fraught with problems. It is almost impossible to exercise proper control over the dosage for one thing, and secondly, some herbs are so unpalatable in their natural state as to make their prescription in this manner rather unpleasant to say the least.

Consequently, it becomes obvious that the desired method of ingesting herbal material is also the least practicable. For this reason herbalists over the centuries have developed alternative ways of giving medicines to patients, and no-one can effectively use herbs for medicinal purposes unless a knowledge of these methods is gained first.

EXTRACTIONS

Simply speaking, an extraction is any herbal medicine that has as

43

its basis the extracted fluid or properties of a plant, but does not contain particles of the actual plant material itself. There are five major methods of producing extractions.

Infusions: Sometimes called tisanes, infusions are the quickest way of producing herbal medicines, and also the simplest. To make a good infusion you will need:

1) A small pan.
2) A measuring jug, preferably glass.
3) A set of household scales.
4) A tea strainer.
5) One ounce of dried herb for every pint of medicine that you require (normally speaking).

Before we discuss the actual method of infusing in any depth, it is important that we first give some consideration to the equipment that we are to use.

The pan should be enamel (or iron as a second choice). NEVER use copper or aluminium pans as they impart a bitter flavour to the herb, and small particles of these metals have been known to find their way into the human digestive system. Enamel and iron have a greater degree of hardness and are generally regarded as acceptable.

A good measuring jug is a necessity. It should be constructed of heat-proof glass, but if this is not available, a good quality 'plus' polymer.

An accurate set of scales is necessary for measuring out quantities of the dried herb. Always check that your scales are properly adjusted before you begin.

The strainer serves a dual purpose. Not only does it carry out the obvious task of removing plant particles from the infusion, but it can also be used to increase the strength of the medicine as we shall see.

Method: Pour one pint of cold water into a pan. (Use bottled mountain or spring water if it is available.) Heat the water to boiling point, switch off the heat and wait for thirty seconds. Then sprinkle the herb into the water and stir. *Never* pour boiling water over the dried herb or add the herb directly to water that is still boiling, as this destroys the potency. Leave the plant material in the water for ten minutes, giving the occasional stir. Then, pour the liquid through the strainer into another receptacle. If a stronger tisane is required, re-pour the liquid through the plant particles in the strainer two or three times.

Those who find the bitter taste of some infusions disagreeable can sweeten them with honey or brown sugar.

Decoctions: The art of preparing a good decoction takes minutes to learn and yet years to master. Made correctly, they are potent medicines that need to be taken only in relatively small amounts. Made incorrectly they are nothing short of useless.

Method: Take one ounce of the dried herb and place it in the bottom of the pan. Add one pint of cold water and slowly bring it to the boil. When the water has reached boiling point, turn down the heat and allow the liquid to boil or simmer down to one quarter of its orginal volume. The decoction should then be strained.

Decoctions are particularly valuable when making medicines from roots or bark, as their active principles cannot normally be drawn out in sufficient quantities simply by making an infusion.

Percolations: To produce a stronger medicine than is normally possible by infusion, some herbalists percolate an ounce of the dried herb in an ordinary, household coffee percolator. This method does have certain advantages, but unless you are experienced in the properties of various herbs it may be wise to seek professional guidance from a colleague. Some plants, particularly those rich in tannins, can cause severe gastric disturbances if they are percolated over a long period of time.

Expressions: The removal of the volatile oils or natural juices of the plant by mechanical means. Volatile oils are often used externally (this practice is called aromatherapy) but some – such as the oil of Garlic (*Allium sativa*) – can be taken internally for a variety of ailments.

Tinctures: Sometimes called macerations. Alcohol is much more effective than water for drawing out the medicinal properties of plants. Because of this many herbalists soak fresh or dried herbs in alcohol for prolonged periods of time. The resultant mixture is an extremely potent medicine that need only be administered in extremely small amounts.

Method: There are various methods used in the manufacture of tinctures, but the simplest way is to soak one ounce of the herb in one

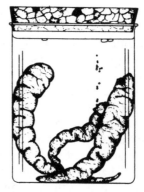

Roots may be stored in alcohol indefinitely to produce tinctures of various strengths.

pint of alcohol for a period of eight weeks. The container should be shaken daily for the first four weeks.

CAUTION: *NEVER* use wood alcohol or methanol as this can be a deadly poison.

OTHER METHODS

Liquid extractions are undoubtedly the most common types of herbal preparation, but there are others. Pills, tablets, poultices and ointments are also often used.

Pills: The art of encapsulating herbal medicines in small pills was first developed by Oriental physicians some 1,800 years B.C. The advantages are numerous, as pills are not only convenient to take but also enable the dosage to be monitored accurately. Unfortunately, pills have a rather short shelf-life, and will last for nine months at the most.

Method: Making pills on a small scale at home is rather tricky, but the following procedure should suffice.

Take ½ ounce of the dried herb and powder finely. Mix this with enough edible gum or gelatine to make a stiff paste, and then coat the mixture with fine icing sugar. The gel should then be carefully rolled into strips that are approximately 2/5 of an inch in thickness. The strips should then be cut themselves at intervals of 2/5 of an inch and then left to harden.

Tablets: The making of tablets on a small scale is not possible without purchasing some rather elaborate – and hideously expensive – equipment. Concentrated extracts are subjected to great pressure and then moulded into shape, dried, and then finally coated with a fine layer of sugar to make them palatable.

Poultices: Less fashionable now than in times past, the poultice is still extremely useful for the treatment of external lesions and ulcers. It is also good for drawing out boils and suppurations. Fresh herbs are normally applied directly to the wound and covered with a sterile bandage.

Suppositories: Suppositories are small rocket-shaped devices that contain liquid extract (or the fine comminution of) a medicinal herb. They are normally made from a sterile hydrogenated fat (that is, a fat that is solid at room temperature) or from some other heat-sensitive material. When they are inserted into the rectal passage the increase in temperature causes them to melt and release the medication into the bowel.

This is ideal if the medicine is intended for some disorder of the large intestine, but as the bowel is constantly absorbing water it can also absorb medication and ensure that it is transported to other parts of the body.

Pessaries: Similar to suppositories, but designed for insertion into the vaginal orifice. Pessaries are normally used in the treatment of vaginal infections and discharges. It is NEVER advisable to use pessaries during pregnancy unless you are advised to do so by a physician or qualified herbalist.

4 Glossary of Medical Terms

ABORTIFACIENT Any herb that induces the spontaneous expulsion of the foetus before it can survive. A deliberate termination of the life within the womb.

ALTERATIVE Any herb which is acknowledged to have the ability to alter a patient's condition from one state to another. A mono-alterative acts in one way only; that is, it is capable of producing an effect – such as raising the blood pressure – but is incapable of producing the opposite effect, in this case *lowering* the blood pressure.

A true alterative is capable of producing both effects, and Ginseng (*Panax quinquefolia*) is a classic example. Some studies have shown that hypertensive (high blood pressure) patients will see a reduction in their blood pressure, whilst hypotensive (low blood pressure) patients will actually see theirs raised.

How this double-barrelled action works is not quite understood, but there is a possibility that an as yet undiscovered body mechanism in some way rejects the active principles that it does not require, whilst absorbing those that it needs. This theory was advanced several years ago, and is admittedly imperfect, but it would seem to explain the curious way in which some herbs produce two opposite effects in different patients.

ANODYNE A herb with pain-killing properties. *Valeriana officinalis* (Valerian) is a good example.

ANTHELMINTIC   Any herb used to aid the expulsion of worms from the intestinal tract. *Brunella vulgaris* (All-Heal), *Melia azadirachta* (Azadirachta) and *Spigela marilandica* (Carolina Pinkroot) are reported by many herbalists to be effective anthelmintics.

ANTHILIC   Any herb that prevents the formation of stones within the urinary tract. *Berberis Linne* (Trailing Mahonia) is quite effective.

ANTIBILIOUS   Any herb used to prevent the excessive production of bile and the unpleasant symptoms of such. The Egyptians have used *Cinnamomum zeylanicum* (Cinnamon) for nearly four thousand years.

ANTIEMETIC   Any herb used to prevent vomiting or the regurgitation of the gastric contents into the oesophagus. *Lobelia inflata* (Padded Lobelia) is an antiemetic when taken in small quantities. However, it will actually induce vomiting if taken in excess.

ANTILEPTIC   Any herb that has the property of reducing morbid fits or seizures. *Convallaria majalis* (Lily of the Valley), *Hyssopus officinalis* (Hyssop) and *Phorandendron flavescens* (Mistletoe) are well known antileptics.

ANTINAUSEANT   Any herb used to prevent the feeling of nausea. *Iris versicolor* (Blue Flag) is recommended.

ANTIPERIODIC   Any herb that prevents the return or the regular reoccurrence of an illness. *Linaria elatine* (Fluelinne) is one example.

ANTISCORBUTENT   A herb used in the prevention of scurvy or some other illness that causes skin delamination. *Taraxacum officinalis* (Dandelion) is one possible choice of many.

ANTISEPTIC — Any herb that prevents tissue degeneration and the formation of puss. *Hamamelis virginiana* (Witch Hazel), *Rubus vilosus* (Blackberry) and *Ribes nigrum* (Black Currant) are examples.

ANTISPASMODIC — Any herb used to treat diseases that are characterized by symptoms of sudden onset such as angina. *Scutellaria lateriflora* (Scullcap) is popular with American practitioners.

APERIENT — Any herb that is mildly laxative in nature, but not as potent as a cathartic. *Taraxacum officinalis* (Dandelion) is the most commonly available aperient in the U.K.

APHRODISIAC — Any herb that facilitates sexual excitement, i.e., causes a physical arousal within the sexual organs through an irritant action, or a strong mental desire to engage in sexual activity. Three proven aphrodisiacs that are used in the treatment of sexual debility are: *Liriosma ovata* (Muira Puama), *Pimenta officinalis* (Allspice) and the skin of *Musa sapientum* (Banana). The latter may be dangerous if taken in excess, and it should be said at this juncture that the taking of aphrodisiacs purely to heighten sexual pleasure is most strongly contraindicated. The use of aphrodisiacs in a medical scenario is also extremely limited.

AROMATIC — Any herb that acts as a stimulant to the digestive organs. *Eugenia aromatica* (Clove) is a good example.

ASTRINGENT — Any herb that draws together or tightens the tissues. Plants rich in tannins are usually astringent. *Viburnum rufidulum* (Stagbush) and *Citrus limon* (Lemon) are noteables, the former being used chiefly in the U.S.A. and the latter in Europe.

BITTER

Any herb that has a bitter but not necessarily unpleasant taste. *Cusparia febrifugia* (Angustura) is a well known bitter often used to flavour alcoholic beverages.

CARDIAC

Any herb that has an effect upon the heart. *Viola tricolor* (Wild Pansy or Heartsease) and *Digitalis pulverata* (Digitalis) are prime examples.

CARMINATIVE

Any herb that assists the expulsion of gas from the intestines or stomach, and not, as has been claimed by some herbalists who should know better, a herb with a sedative action! *Nepeta cataria* (Catnip) is excellent for this purpose.

CATHARTIC

A powerful laxative that promotes an extremely quick evacuation of the bowels. *Ferula foetiola Regel* (Asafoetida or Devil's Dung) and *Polymnia uvedalia* (American Bearsfoot) are examples.

CEPHALIC

Any herb used to treat diseases of the brain.

CHOLAGOGUE

Any herb that increases or promotes bile production. *Symphytum officinale* (Comfrey) has been recommended.

DEMULCENT

Any herb that soothes and lubricates the intestines. *Ulmus fulva* (Slippery Elm) is perhaps the most widely known herbal demulcent. Stomach ulcers and other gastric disorders often respond well to this marvellous plant remedy.

DEOBSTRUENT

Any herb with laxative properties.

DEPURATIVE

Any herb that purifies the blood. *Allium sativa* (Garlic) is probably the most widely used depurative amongst British and European herbalists.

DETERGENT

Any herb with antiseptic properties, but normally used to cleanse the skin. The Blackfoot and Apache indians made great use of *Trillium pendulum* (Bethroot) to treat arrow and gunshot wounds. Studies carried out by the Institute of Plant Medicines Research indicate that the antiseptic and detergent properties of *T. pendulum* have not been overestimated.

DIAPHORETIC   Any herb that increases bodily perspiration. Several plants, such as *Valeriana officinalis* (Valerian) induce heavy sweating or diaphoresis, but this is often due to their toxicity when taken in excess. Herbs that induce perspiration naturally include *Aristolochia serpentaria* (Snakeroot), *Smilax aristolochioefolia* (Sarsaparilla), *Sassafras officinalis* (Sassafras), *Calendula officinalis* (Marigold) and *Macrotys actaeoides* (Square Root).

DIGESTRON   A special technique used in the production of strong macerations or tinctures.

DIURETIC   Herbs that promote or induce urination, of which *Taraxacum officinalis* (Dandelion) is probably the most interesting example. The different varieties of *T. officinalis* are often called 'wet-the-beds' because the powerful diuretic chemicals within the stem can be absorbed through the skin, and often cause nocturnal enuresis (bedwetting) in young children who handle the plant on a regular basis.

EMETIC   Any herb used to induce vomiting. Some emetics, such as *Strychnos nux-vomica* (Poison Nut or Quakers' Buttons), are extremely poisonous even in small amounts, and their use is rarely – if ever – justified.

EMMENAGOGUE   Any herb used to promote the menstrual flow, including *Solanum dulcamara* (Bittersweet) and *Anthemis nobilis* (Chamomile).

EMOLIENT   Any herb with skin-soothing properties. *Popu-*

lus candicans (Balm Of Gilead) is an excellent emolient, but whether this is the Balm Of Gilead mentioned in the Holy Bible has long been a matter of dispute.

EXANTHEMATE A herbal remedy that is used in the treatment of skin eruptions.

EXPECTORANT Any herb that facilitates the removal of excess mucous from the bronchial tubes. *Zingiber officinale* (Ginger), *Lonicera caprifolium* (Honeysuckle) and *Marrubium vulgare* (Hoar Hound) are examples.

FEBRIFUGE Any herb that reduces an unusually high body temperature. *Berberis aristata* (Indian Berberis) and *Hydrastis canadensis* (Goldenseal) are popular in this regard along with others such as *Crysanthemum parthenium* (Feverfew), *Gentiana lurea* (Gentain) and *Aegle marmelos* (Bengal Quince).

HAEMOSTATIC Any herb used to arrest bleeding or promote blood-clotting. A surprising number of medicinal herbs have this property. Some, such as *Pinus palustris* (Turpentine) and *Plantago major* (Plantain), are used chiefly for the prevention of external bleeding, whilst some, such as *Trillium pendulum* (Beth Root), can be used to treat both internal and external bleeding.

Strangely, some plants seem to have the peculiar property of arresting bleeding in one group of organs only. *Linaria elatine* (Fluelinne) is remarkably effective at reducing bleeding from the ear, nose and throat, but it's ability to arrest bleeding elsewhere in the body appears to be only marginal.

HEPATIC Any herb that stimulates or aids the function of the liver or gall-bladder.

HERPATIC   See Exanthemous.

HYPNOTIC   Any herb that induces drowsiness, sleep or a trance-like state within the patient. NEVER take any plant with hypnotic qualities unless it is under medical supervision. Hypnotics are not to be confused with sedatives.

IRRITANT   Any herb that produces pain, itchiness or swellings on contact with the skin, or alternatively, any plant that generates sexual excitement when applied externally to the genital organs or taken internally.

LAXATIVE   Any herb that induces bowel evacuation.

LYTHONTRYPTIC   Any plant that encourages the catabolism or breakdown of urinary stones or calculii. *Agropyron repens* (Couchgrass) and any of the *vetis* (Grape) genera are useful for this purpose.

MYDRIATIC   Any herb that increases the size of the pupil of the eye. Mydriatic herbs such as *Atropa belladonna* (Deadly Nightshade) were highly favoured by Egyptian and Babylonian noblewomen who dropped small amounts of the liquid extract into their eyes, thus making themselves more attractive to prospective suitors.

MYOTIC   Any herb that possesses the ability to constrict the pupil of the eye.

NATURANT   A herb that is a good 'drawing' medium and can bring 'blind' spots or boils to a head thus creating a natural apex through which putrative matter can be expelled. The most efficient naturant – but one which has fallen into disuse in the West – is *Ficus carica* (Fig). The bible records its use by Isaiah the Prophet (2nd Kings ch. 20) in healing King Hezekiah of a boil which had become septic and threatened to kill him.

NAUSEANT   Same meaning as antinauseant.

NERVINE   Any herb that allays or remedies nervous disorders. There are a large number of herbs that fall into this category, including mild sedatives and powerful hypnotics. Some, such as *Arthemis nobilis* (Chamomile), seem to have a more beneficial effect on women, whilst others like *Passiflora incranata* (Passion Flower) work equally as well with males.

OPTHALMICUM   Any herb regarded as being of benefit to the eyes. *Euphrasia officinalis* (Eyebright) is held in particularly high esteem by many practitioners.

PARASITICIDE   A plant that is useful for the removal of parasites. African *pyrethrum* is often used in commercial pesticides.

PARTURIENT   Any herb that hastens or initiates the onset of parturition or birth. There is no real difference between a parturient and an abortifacient other than in the dosage given and the time at which it is taken. It goes without saying that NO herbal or other parturient should be taken to initiate labour except under strict medical supervision.

PECTORAL   Any herbal remedy for chest infections.

PURGATIVE   A powerful laxative. *Prinos verticillatus* (Black Alder), *Fraxinus excelsior* (European Ash) and *Asplenium scolopendrium* (Hart's Tongue) are some examples.

REFRIGERANT   Similar to an emolient but being particularly useful for the treatment of burns and rashes. Many herbalists use *Acacia arabica* (Gum Arabic).

RESOLVENT   Dissolves boils and tumours. Often called a discutient.

RUBIFACIENT   Any herb that increases the flow of blood to the skin, or irritates the skin in any manner, both of which result in a flush of colour to the cheeks. Ancient civilizations prized rubifacient herbs highly before the advent of modern cosmetics.

SEDATIVE

Any herb that has the ability to induce restful sleep or a feeling of calmness within the patient. *Borago officinalis* (Borage) and *Passiflora incranata* (Passion Flower) are often used to accomplish this.

SIALOGOGUE

Any herbal medicine that induces the flow of saliva. *Carum carvi* (Caraway) is a popular culinary sialogogue.

SIMPLE

Any herbal medicine that is made from one herb only, as compared to compound remedies that are made from two or more herbs.

STERNUTATORY

Any herb that causes sneezing when in contact with the nasal passages. All sternutatories are irritants. *Quillaja saponaria* (Soap Tree) is an effective sternutatory when ground into a fine powder.

STIMULANT

Any herb which a) increases the flow of adrenalin, b) increases the body's basal metabolic rate, or c) stimulates the production of digestive juices.

STOMATIC

Sometimes called stomachics, stomatics are herbs that relieve the symptoms of one or more gastric disorders. *Prunus laurocerasus* (Cherry Laurel) and *Cinnamomum zeylanicum* (Cinnamon) are recommended.

STYPTIC

Same as haemostatic.

SUDORIFIC

Same as diaphoretic.

TONIC

Any herbal medicine that has restorative powers and acts as both a stimulant and an alterative to the body. Perhaps the most prized tonic is the Oriental *Panax quinquefolia* or Ginseng.

VERMIFUGE   Same as anthelmintic.

VULNERARY   Any herb that has both styptic *and* antiseptic properties.

PART TWO

1 Naming and Identifying Medicinal Plants

Over the centuries several attempts have been made to categorize the various families, genera and species of plants, but none has ever been adopted on a worldwide basis other than that which is used almost universally today. This method of classifying plant life was developed by the eminent Swedish botanist Carl Linnaeus, or as he is sometimes called, Carl Linne.

In 1753, at the age of forty six, Linnaeus produced one of the outstanding botanical works of all time entitled *Linnaeus on Species Plantarum*. In this work he organized the basic divisions into which plant life is divided. Of course, the science of taxonomy, or the naming of plants, has been somewhat expanded upon since the days of Carl Linnaeus, and if we are to look at the basic divisions of the Plantae Kingdom the best place to start, metaphorically speaking, is at the top.

There are four main divisions in the plant world. These are the Thallophytes, the Bryophytes, the Pteridophytes and the Spermatophytes.

Thallophyta The *Thallophyta* contain approximately (very approximately) 120,000 species. They are simple plants that do not have specific organs that accomplish a certain task or set of tasks. They possess no true roots; they are leafless; they do not flower and they cannot produce seeds.

The Thallophyta contain the simplest forms of plant life that we know, and this group is itself divided into three sub-divisions; the *algae*, the *fungi* and the *bacteria*.

Some botanists question whether the bacteria should really be classed as plant life at all as their structure is so primitive and they contain no chlorophyll.

Bryophyta In this division we begin to see the first real 'plants' in the accepted sense of the word. Although their structure is still quite primitive, bryophytes do possess crude leaf and stem structures. They do not, however, possess true roots. The *Bryophyta* are the second smallest of the four main groups (about 20,000 species) and are themselves divided into two sub-divisions; the Mosses and the Liverworts.

Pteridophyta   The smallest order of plants. They are still quite primitive in structure but do possess true root systems. The three sub-divisions of Pteriodphyta are Ferns, Horsetails and Clubmosses.

Spermatophyta   This is the fourth group and the one that is most important to man. Spermatophyta are divided into two sub-divisions. They are the Gymnosperms and the Angiosperms. The gymnosperms contain the evergreens, Larches, Conifers, Pines etc; plants that generally grow to be of considerable size and that possess woody stems.

The angiosperms contain all the flowering plants and trees and also the main vegetable crops such as the cabbage and potato.

But of course, we know that not all flowers are the same, in just the same way that we know that not all vegetables are the same. And so we must break down these groups even further to assist classification. After the sub-divisions, the next sub-grouping is that of the Family.

A family is a group of plants within the same order or sub-order that share similar characteristics. Let's take a look at one example:

Within the Angiospermal group there is a family known as the *Liliaceae*. These are plants that possess swollen, underground or creeping stems and unbranched, short-stalked flowers. They also produce berries or capsulous fruits. There are thousands of species within the *Liliaceae* Family, and these can be classified even further. For instance, there are nearly one hundred species of a flower known as the Lily within the *Liliaceae* Family; but *Liliaceae* also contains another group of plants (*Allium*) which include the Onion and Garlic. Now no-one would suggest that the Lily (whatever species) is usually spoken of as synonymous with Garlic or Onion, and so to separate the various kinds of plant within the *Lilaceae* family botanists have grouped them down into further sections. Within every family of the plant kingdom there are also *genera*.

A *genus* is a sub-division of a Family. The aforementioned flowers called Lilies are grouped together under the *Lilium* genus, whilst the Onion and Garlic are part of the *Allium* genus. Both genera are part of the *Liliaceae* Family.

So we have established that the Onion and Garlic are part of the *Liliaceae* Family, which in turn belongs to a sub-division of the spermatophytes known as the angiosperms. But our system of classification must be taken further, because everyone knows that Garlic and Onion – although similar – are *not* the same plant. Linnaeus thus added a secondary or 'Christian' name if you like, that would enable botanists to differentiate between two different species. That is why the Onion is called *Allium cepa* and Garlic is called *Allium sativum*.

Now this system is fine as far as it goes, but what happens when a person wishes to describe a certain type of species? For instance, if I went into a supermarket and asked for a pound of apples, the assistant would likely ask me 'What kind of apples? Cox's Pippins? Golden Delicious? Granny Smith's?' These are all members of the apple species, and yet they are different.

This last distinction – variance within a species – is denoted by the word variety. Thus, if one wanted to describe a Golden Delicious apple botanically, the correct term would be *Malus* (genus) *pumila* (species) var. Golden Delicious.

The chart traces the botanical pedigree of the Onion by way of an example.

THE USE OF COMMON NAMES

One other important point needs to be stressed before we close this chapter. Although it is far easier to use common names when talking about various herbs (seriously, who would keep saying *Smilax aristolochioefolia* when they could get away with Sarsaparilla?), it is dangerous to fall into the trap of *never* using the botanical name. Some common names can be applied to totally different species. In some parts of the U.S.A. Sarsaparilla is commonly called Bittersweet. The name Bittersweet, however, is also applied to the deadly poisonous *Solanum dulcamara*. You don't

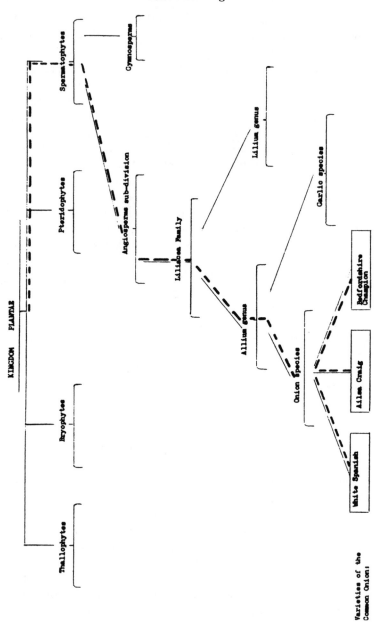

KINGDOM   PLANTAE

Thallophytes
Bryophytes
Pteridophytes
Spermatophytes

Gymnosperms
Angiosperms sub-division

Liliaceae Family

Lilium genus
Garlic species
Allium genus

Onion Species

Bedfordshire Champion
Ailsa Craig
White Spanish

Varieties of the
Common Onion:

have to be a genius to consider the disastrous consequences of mistaking one for the other.

If you are ordering herbs from a supplier, ALWAYS quote the correct botanical name in your order.

2   A Concise Herbal

INTRODUCTION

Administering the correct dosage of a herbal medicine is perhaps one of the most knotty problems that the herbalist can face, particularly if he makes up his own medicines. Appendix 1 gives a general guide as to the proportionate dosages, but other factors, such as the varying amounts of active principles in different species and varieties of the same plant, must also be taken into consideration.

Often, the reader will be told that a tisane should be made at 'Standard Strength'. This refers to the standard British method of adding one ounce of the dried herb to one pint of water. For further details see the chapter on *Making Herbal Medicines*.

- **ABCESS ROOT**   *Polemonium reptans*
Botanical information: This plant, which belongs to the *Polemoniaceae* family, grows prolifically in Scandinavian countries and is characterized by the clusters of delicate, wire-like roots that grow from the lower surface of the rhizome.

Therapeutic uses: *P. reptans* is used almost exclusively in the treatment of pulmonary diseases, and an examination of the herb's various medicinal properties clearly shows why.

P. reptans is, even in moderate doses, a powerful diaphoretic, and will cause profuse sweating in the patient. The advantages of this in those conditions that are accompanied by a fever are obvious, and the temperature should begin to drop after one or two doses.

The herb is also an astringent and antiseptic, and will soothe an inflamed bronchial mucosa and promote the rapid healing of an ulcerated throat.

Perhaps the most valuable aspect of this herb's medicinal qualities is its use as an expectorant. It will quickly remove mucous from the lungs and bronchi, and as the herb also produces a slight vasodilative action it makes breathing easier and reduces coughing.

The herb is more popular in the U.S.A. than in Great Britain, and American herbalists seem particularly intrigued by its alterative properties.

It is also said that a tincture of the herb painted on brittle nails *ad lib* will strengthen them.

Dosage: Tisane, Standard Strength. Two fl oz to be taken twice a day, hot.

Synonyms: American Greek Valerian, False Jacob's Ladder, Sweatroot, Abscess Plant.

- **ACACIA** *Acacia senegal*

Botanical information: A large genus of evergreens belonging to the *Leguminosae* family, which comprises of over 800 species. Africa, the Middle East and Australia play host to the most popular species, all of which have various medicinal properties.

Therapeutic Uses: *A. senegal* is valued for the gummy exudate which collects on the surface of its branches. The gum was applied to loose teeth by the ancient Egyptians, and with good reason. It's thick, mucilaginous qualities helped to support the tooth, whilst it's astringent qualities tightened up the surrounding gum tissue. If the damage was not too severe, the tooth would often 'firm-up' in a short space of time.

The gum was also applied to open wounds as an antiseptic balm.

The African *A. catechu* and the Australian *A. pycnantha* both have tannin-rich bark, and a decoction of it can be applied to inflamed tissue and burns to promote rapid healing and a knitting together of the tissues.

This high tannin content has also caused the herb to be used in the treatment of mouth ulcers and throat inflammation. It's astringency helps check the growth of oral bacteria and soothes the delicate tissues that line the inside of the mouth.

Dosage: As directed by a physician or qualified herbalist. Some species can be used internally in the treatment of various digestive disorders, but the tannic acid content may be so high that, far from promoting a healing action, the gastric mucosa may be severely irritated.

Synonyms: Gum Arabic, Acacia Gum, Egyptian Thorn, Wattle, Black Catechu, Tamerisk, Tamarisk, Senegal Gum, Babul.

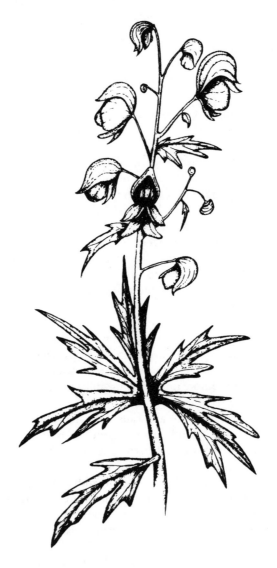

ACONITE (*Aconitum napellus*) is a poisonous herb used in small amounts to treat the symptoms of Parkinsonism

- **ACONITE** *Aconitum napellus*

Botanical information: *Aconitum* is a large genus of perennials native to Europe, North America and some parts of Southern and Central Asia. The Aconites belong to the *Ranunculaceae* family of which there are between 300 – 350 species.

It must be said at this juncture that ALL species of this group contain, to a greater or lesser degree, the deadly poisonous alkaloids *Aconitine* and *Pseudoaconitine,* and if they are accidentally ingested in anything more than microscopic quantities the consequences will invariably be fatal. There is no really effective cure for Aconite poisoning, although John Gerard refers to one in his *Herbal Or General History Of Plants.*

Therapeutic uses: Aconite can only be described as a medicinal herb if it is taken in minute quantities. It will regulate the heartbeat, reduce nervous tension, and may temporarily relieve the symptoms of Parkinson's Disease.

The herb has been employed as a febrifuge and has also been employed in times past, with varying degrees of success, in the treatment of scarlet fever, croup and thrush.

Dosage: None can be safely recommended.

Synonyms: Black Sea Root, Wolfsbane, Wolf's Bane, Aconis, Monkshood, Friar's Mantle, Blue Rocket, Thora, Bastard Aconite.

- **AGAR-AGAR** *Gelidium amansii*

Botanical information: *Gelidium* is a genus of algae which belongs to the *Gelidaceae* family. It grows prolifically in the China Seas and all around the Asiatic Coast.

The refining of Agar-Agar is a complex process. In the summer the algae is spread out to dry in the sun. When thoroughly bleached, the dried herb is boiled in pure water which soon turns into a thick gummy liquid. The liquid is then separated from the waste by straining.

When cool, the liquid solidifies and is cut into thin strips. These are then dried and stored in a cool place to prevent the growth of mould. The product is then ground down into a fine powder which is then ready for both commercial and medicinal use.

Therapeutic uses: Traditionally, *G. amansii* is made into a jelly and given to the sick and infirm. It is an excellent foodstuff because of its high protein content.

The herb is also mildly laxative and will gently evacuate the bowels without purging.

Dosage: The jelly can be given in moderate quantities just like any other foodstuff, but excessive amounts may cause flatulence and slight diarrhoea.

Synonyms: Agar, Agar Weed, Japanese Isinglass.

● **ALSTONIA BARK**   *Alstonia constricta*

Botanical information: *A. constricta*, the more popular of the two main species, is a native of Australia and is used extensively by the Aborigines as a folk-remedy. *A. scholaris* is also used medicinally, but grows more prolifically in India, Pakistan and the Philippines.

Therapeutic uses: Alstonia bark is used almost exclusively as a febrifuge, and those herbalists who have had experience of it normally agree that there is no finer medium for reducing the temperature of a febrile patient. The herb also has some popularity in Australia and New Zealand as a cure for rheumatism.

Outside Australia, its use as a medicine seems more highly appreciated in the U.S.A. than anywhere else, but it is gaining a mention in British Herbals with increasing frequency.

Dosage: Both English authorities (Wren, R.C., *Potter's New Cyclopaedia Of Botanical Drugs and Preparations*, Health Science Press, 1971.) and American authorities (Kadans, Joseph., *Modern Encyclopaedia of Herbs*, Parker Publishing Company, 1970.) recommend a dosage of 2–8 grains, this of course depending on the age and condition of the patient. The powdered bark, in the amount mentioned above, should be made into a tisane and drunk whilst hot.

Synonyms: Australian Quinine, Australian Fever Bark.

● **ANGELICA**   *Angelica archangelica*

Botanical information: The Angelicas, a genus of around 60 species that are part of the *Umbelliferae* family, grow in the Northern temperate regions and seem to thrive particularly well in New Zealand. The cultivated varieties have extremely thick rhizomes, whilst the wild angelicas sport thin conical roots.

Therepeutic uses: Those who are more versed in the culinary uses of herbs as opposed to their medicinal ones will probably know Angelica as an aromatic flavouring added to cakes and confectionaries, but the herb also has several therapeutic properties.

A. angelica is a good aid to those who have digestive problems, and is a highly recommended carminative. It will quickly expel gas from the gut and bowel, and may be used with confidence on children as it produces a very gentle action.

The herb also has a reputation as an effective treatment for bladder infection. This can be explained chemically, as the plant possesses antiseptic agents and is also mildy diuretic. The increased flow of urine prevents the build-up of harmful bacteria on the bladder wall. It's antiseptic properties were noted by Gerard who said:

> The root of garden Angelica is a singular remedy against poyson, and against the plague, and all infections taken by evil and corrupt aire.

During the Middle Ages the liquid extract of Angelica was dropped into the eyes and ears of soldiers going into battle in the belief that it would improve their sight and hearing dramatically. Some modern herbalists still prescribe Angelica drops for eye problems, apparently with some success.

Dosage: 25 grains of the powdered root.

Synonyms: Garden Angelica, Angel Root.

- **ANISE SEED** *Pimpinella Anisum*

Botanical information: An annual umbelliferous plant that originated in the orient but can now be found growing throughout Europe and the United States as well as in other places.

Therapeutic uses: Anise Seed (or Aniseed) has a long history as a medicinal herb, gaining a mention in Egyptian papyrii dated to 2,000 B.C.

The herb is generally taken to relieve stomach cramps and other digestive disturbances. It stimulates the flow of digestive juices in the stomach and intestines, and increases the efficiency with which fats are broken down into fatty acids. Besides this, the herb is also a remarkable carminative and will expel wind from the large intestine, particularly if taken in conjunction with *Carum carvi* (Caraway).

A weak tisane (½ tsp of ground Anise Seed to 1 pint of water) also makes a soothing eyewash.

Dosage: As a treatment for digestive disorders and colic, 1 tbsp of ground Anise Seed should be boiled in ½ pint of milk and drunk twice a day.

Synonyms: Star Anise, Aniseed, Annissamen, Anise Cultivé.

● **BALM OF GILEAD**   *Populus candicans*

Botanical information: A small shrub that grows profusely in certain areas of the Middle East, especially around Mecca. (Arabian physicians of old such as Mesu, Rhazes and Avicenna were highly impressed by its medicinal qualities.)

Despite claims to the contrary, their is little evidence to support the idea that *P. candicans* is the Balm of Gilead mentioned in the Bible. In fact, *Pistacia lentiscus* is a far more likely candidate.

The buds, which are the parts used for medicinal purposes, are best collected in late winter.

Therapeutic uses: The oils contained in *P. candicans* are volatile and are readily absorbed through the skin. Their antibiotic and febrifugic qualities make the herb an ideal remedy for chest infections of every kind, and it seems that the duration of colds and some minor strains of influenza can be shortened by the application of Balm of Gilead ointment or lotion to the chest area.

The herb is also useful for the treatment of chronic skin ulcers and other infected wounds. Miller said that the herb was even superior to the turpentines for it's antiseptic properties.

Dosage: The herb can be used as an ingredient in cough syrups, but a dosage of no more than ten grains in twenty-four hours should be needed.

Synonyms: Balsam Poplar, Mecca Balsam, Tacamahack.

● **BELLADONNA**   *Atropa belladonna*

Botanical information: Belladonna (or Deadly Nightshade) is a species of the *Solanaceae* family, and is one of the more notorious plant poisons. It can be found throughout Central and Southern Europe, but in England it only grows in any abundance in the Southern Counties. The plant also grows in certain areas of India and Pakistan.

Therapeutic uses: The first recorded uses of Belladonna are more cosmetic than therapeutic. Egyptian and Babylonian noblewomen would drop a diluted expression of the plant into their eyes to artificially enlarge their pupils. This of course made them subtly more attractive to prospective suitors.

Despite it's poisonous nature – it contains the poisonous alkaloid *hysoscyamine* – *A. belladonna* contains some therapeutic agents also. In

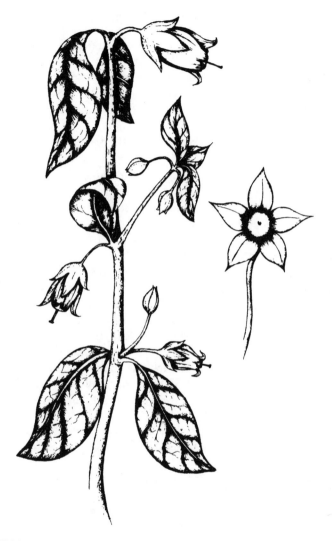

DEADLY NIGHTSHADE (*Atropa belladonna*). Once used as an eye dilator to improve the appearance of Babylonian noblewomen, the herb is now used to treat nervous disorders.

small quantities it proves itself an effective sedative and can be used in the treatment of nervous disorders and hysterical seizures. *A. belladonna* is a febrifuge, and also reduces glandular activity. It has been used with some success in the treatment of spermatorrhoea: an involuntary discharge of semen from the penis.

Dosages: None can be safely recommended to the untrained person. Only QUALIFIED herbalists should prescribe the herb when such is required.

Synonyms: Dwale, Deadly Nightshade, Black Cherry Root.

● **BILBERRY**   *Vaccinium myrtillus*

Botanical information: *V. myrtillus* is common throughout the British Isles and most of Europe, although it cannot be found in Greece or the Atlas Mountains of Morocco. It enjoys damp, boggy soil with a strong acid bias, and can be found in woods, forests and hedgerows. It also inhabits some exposed moorland and heath.

The leaves are best collected in July.

Therapeutic uses: The fruits are an excellent foodstuff and are useful in cases of diarrhoea and bowel inflammation because of their astringent quality. Up to 10% of the liquid extract can be made up of astringent tannins. The berries, if eaten, will solidify the faecal matter and yet not cause constipation. If taken in conjunction with Slippery Elm its soothing action in the bowel is intensified.

Because the plant is rich in Victamin C it has been used in the treatment of scurvy in some Scandinavian countries, and its iron content, 8mg per 100gms, has also proved useful in the treatment of anaemia.

Dosage: The fruit may be eaten ad-lib, but within the normal bounds of moderation. The dried (or fresh) fruit can be made into a tisane at Standard Strength.

Synonyms: Huckleberry, Whortleberry, Hurtleberry.

● **BLUE FLAG**   *Iris versicolor*

Botanical information: A member of the *Iridaceae* family that grows throughout the British Isles. *I. versicolor* is a common garden plant that flowers throughout May and June.

Therapeutic uses: Blue Flag has a variety of medicinal uses, none of which has received sufficient documentation.

Blue Flag is an alterative that can stimulte a sluggish liver into action, and also rid the body of excess fluid accumulations. It has a powerful cathartic action and can remove stubborn cases of constipation. The alkaloids in the rhizome can stimulate heart activity and seem to have a purifying action in the blood. It has been said that the herb may be useful in cases of leukaemia, but I know of no scientific evidence to back up this claim.

The acrid chemicals found in the root were inhaled in liquid form in times past to clear the brain of 'phlegmatic humours'; not a practice that I approve of.

Dosage: No more than 15 grains to be taken by an adult in 24 hours due to its powerful cathartic action. Best left to the experienced practitioner, I would not recommend that this herb be used by the lay practitioner or amateur herbalist.

Synonyms: Poison Flag, Poison Lily, Blue Lily.

● **BORAGE** *Borago officinalis*
Botanical information: An annual plant of the *Boraginaceae* family that is now naturalized to most of Europe, although it is indigenous to the Mediterranean area. Borage is a robust herb that flowers between the months of May and September. It does not require nutrient-rich soil, and can even be grown indoors provided it receives a generous amount of sunlight.

Therapeutic uses: Almost exclusively, Borage is used as a nervine and sedative. The ancient Celts would steep Borage leaves in wine, and the resultant mixture caused a significant rise in the blood–adrenalin level when drunk. This produced something akin to the 'fight or flight' syndrome, except with the Celts it seemed to be all fight and no flight!

Today the herb is added to commercial preparations for the relief of nervous tension, but Borage Tea is still a popular remedy for disorders of this kind. A tisane made from Borage leaves is not unpleasant to take, and once the taste is acquired it may become a person's favourite beverage, although I would not recommend that it be taken too frequently.

Dosage: As a vegetable the leaves can be eaten ad-lib. A tisane can be made to Standard Strength. The liquid expression can be taken ½ dr. every 12 hours.

Synonyms: Borrage, Burrage.

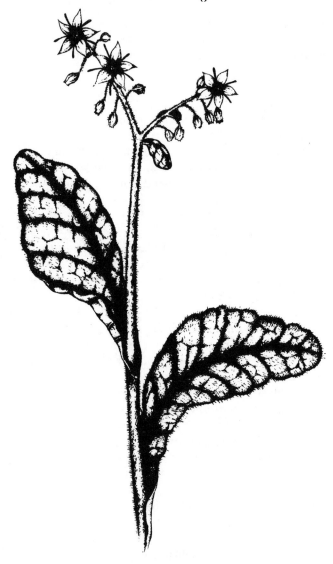

BORAGE (*Borago officinalis*) is one of the most fascinating medical herbs. It has been used since ancient times to treat anxiety states.

- **CARAWAY** *Carum carvi*
Botanical information: A biennial plant of the *Umbelliferae* family. It can be found throughout Europe and North Africa and is cultivated for its aromatic fruits (often called seeds, but wrongly so).

English Caraway is of excellent quality, being viewed by most as superior to the Dutch and African varieties. Caraway only grows wild in a few areas of Britain, but it is cultivated extensively on a cottage level.

Therapeutic uses: Caraway has two principle functions in the practice of botanic medicine. It is an excellent carminative and is the premier medicine of choice for those troubled by gas in the digestive tract. Also, it is a powerful appetite stimulant and can be valuable in cases of endogenous anorexia. Tyneside herbalist Harry Eagles was adept at using this herb in the treatment of digestive disorders, and was probably the country's leading expert on it's therapeutic virtues. He used a personally developed formula for producing tincture of Caraway, and many of his patients still testify to it's efficacy in treating serious cases of anorexia.

Dosage: Tincture of Caraway should be taken in 6 minim amounts.

Synonyms: Alcaravea, Carryways, Carrywa.

- **CATNIP** *Nepeta cataria*
Botanical information: N. cataria is a mint species of the *Labiatae* family which grows throughout the U.K. but is found in greatest abundance in the South East of England. It flowers in late June/July, and should be picked then if possible.

Therapeutic uses: Catnip has antiseptic properties and can be used in poultice form to treat scabs, boils and other skin lesions. A shampoo made from a tisane of the herb can be used to treat dandruff, and it can also be applied to acne pimples as a lotion.

Internally, Catnip may be taken for stomach cramps and indigestion by way of a tisane.

Gerard says that the herb taken 'with wine or meade' is good for those that 'be bursten inwardly of some fall received from an high place'.

Dosage: An infusion of Standard Strength.

Synonyms: Catnep, Catmint, Nep, Herb Catta.

- **CHAMOMILE** *Anthemis nobilis*
Botanical information: *A. nobilis* is a perennial herb of the *Compositae*

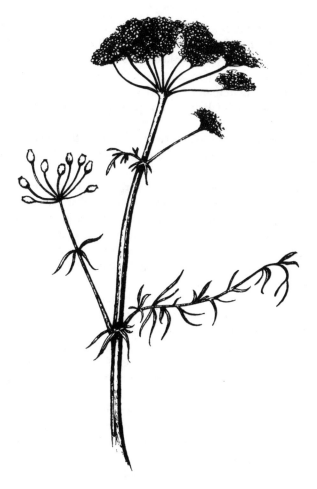

CARAWAY (*Carum carvi*). A popular herbal remedy for digestive disorders that has been in use for nearly four thousand years.

family that flowers from June to September. It is indigenous to Western Europe and grows in large quantities in Belgium, Italy and France. The herb is not cultivated in the U.K. to any great extent, – although Roman Chamomile (*Matricaria chamomilla*) is, but in recent years it has been seen with increasing frequency in rocky areas and pastures.

Therapeutic uses: The primary medicinal use for chamomile in mainland Europe – particularly Italy – is in the treatment of digestive disorders. The flavonoid glycosides combined with the bitter principles in the herb produce an anti-inflammatory effect which soothes the delicate mucous membranes in the stomach.

In the U.K. particular interest has been shown in using *A. nobilis* to treat the symptoms of pre-menstrual tension. The plant also has several organic anodynes present in the flowerheads which help to relieve cramps in the lower abdomen, a common symptom of PMT.

Dosage: A tisane of Standard Strength should be taken three times a day.

Synonyms: Sailors Buttons, Double Chamomile, Camomile, Camomille.

- **CHICKWEED** *Stellaria media*

Botanical information: Chickweed is a weak annual that flowers all the year round. It is a member of the *Caryophyllaceae* family and grows in abundance throughout the entire British Isles and Western Europe. It seems to thrive in areas where cultivation of the land is commonplace, but in areas where farming is abandoned the herb will dwindle and become rather scarce. The plant also thrives in unattended gardens and allotments.

Therapeutic uses: Chickweed is no longer as popular as in times past for it's medicinal uses, but it still carries a reputation as a good skin tonic, particularly in the South of England. The liquid expression is useful for soothing keens, sores and scaly or itchy patches, and two or three pounds of the fresh herb placed in a hot bath will tone up and invigorate the skin.

S. media is also good for certain kidney disorders as it has diuretic properties, but caution should be exercised. An excessive dose can have an untoward effect upon kidney function, and, in rare cases, has caused heart failure.

Dosage: A tisane should be made to standard strength, but no more than 8 fl. oz. should be taken in 24 hrs. Prolonged use should be medically supervised.

Synonyms: Starweed, Star Chickweed.

- **COLTSFOOT**   *Tussilago farfara*

Botanical information: A perennial herb of the *Compositae* family that is to be found throughout Europe, the U.K., North West Africa, Asia and the U.S.A. It inhabits damp, clay-rich soil and arable land and will grow just as happily in an urban environment as in the country. It is a pioneering plant that will quickly inhabit new areas suitable for growth before other plants can become established. It flowers during April and May.

Therapeutic uses: *T. farfara* is now used almost exclusively in the treatment of bronchial and pulmonary disorders. The Amerindians have used Coltsfoot as a medicine for over two-thousand years, placing considerable value on it's curative properties in cases of coughs, colds, lung diseases and also skin ailments.

The plant mucilagens have a soothing effect upon the bronchi and will protect the delicate mucous membranes from further irritation. Coltsfoot is also rich in tannins, which, because of their astringent nature, promote rapid tissue healing.

The use of Coltsfoot in the treatment of skin diseases is greeted with varying degrees of enthusiasm. Some authorities point to it's long history as an emollient and refrigerant in folk-medicine lore, whilst others – rather less than impressed by the results of some clinical trials – feel that it's efficacy in this regard is at best weak.

Dosage: A decoction can be made by decocting 1 qt. of water down to 2/3 of a pint, using 1 oz. of the dried herb. The dosage, in the case of coughs, is one or two teasponfuls as required.

Synonyms: Coughwort, Horsehoof, Horse Hoof, Cough Herb, Foal's Foot, Fool's Foot.

- **DANDELION**   *Taraxacum officinalis*

Botanical information: The Dandelion is a perennial herb and a member of the *Compositae* family. It is found in almost every country of the world, but in particular abundance in the British isles, Western and Central Europe and the U.S.A.

Therapeutic uses: The Dandelion is probably the most widely distributed (and possibly the most widely used) of all medical herbs. It is also true to say that were it as rare as Ginseng, it would undoubtedly command a similar price.

Dandelions have gained a deserved notoriety because of their diuretic properties, which are often absorbed through the skin of

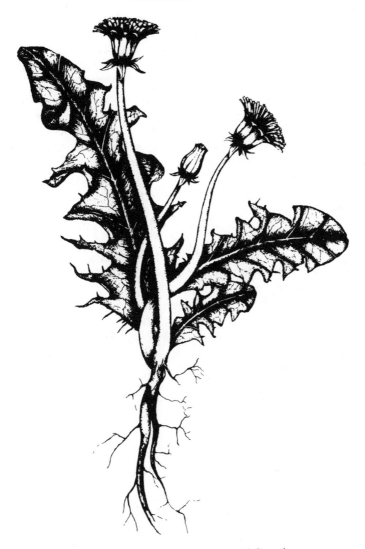

DANDELION (*Taraxacum officinale*) is a powerful diuretic.

young children who handle the flowers too much. If they are fondled regularly, enough diuretic material may be absorbed through the skin to cause nocturnal enuresis or bed-wetting. The diuretic properties of *T. officinalis* were recognized long before the active principles were discovered and chemically isolated, hence the old common name 'Wet-the-Beds'. This diuretic ability has caused the Dandelion to be used successfully in the treatment of several kidney ailments and also chronic hypertension.

Dandelion greens are extremely nutritious. They contain an incredible 13,650 I.U.s of Vitamin A per 100 gms, a generous smattering of the B vitamins and also 36 mg. of Vitamin C.

Claims that *T. officinalis* can arrest the growth of certain types of malignant tumour have not been attested to by the American National Cancer Institute, and reports concerning it's efficacy in the treatment of eczema also seem to be exaggerated.

Dosage: A tisane can be made to Standard Strength, and taken three times a day, one cupful at a time. The leaves can be eaten as a vegetable.

Synonyms: Taraxacum, Lion's Tooth, Puff-Ball, Swine Snout, Wild Endive, Blow-Ball, Priest's crown, Sun In The Grass.

● **ELDER** *Sambucus nigra*

Botanical information: The European or Common Elder (*S. nigra*) and it's North American cousin *S. canadensis* (American or Sweet Elder) are both popular garden trees. They inhabit temperate and sub-tropical countries, and the berries ripen in September when they should be picked for use.

Therapeutic uses: Both the two main species of Elder mentioned above, and also to a lesser extent *S. ebulus* (Dane's or Viking Elder), are used for medicinal purposes. They are all midly diaphoretic, and are used to alleviate the symptoms of colds and influenza when taken as a tisane. This restorative action is enhanced if the herb is taken with *Mentha piperita* (Peppermint).

The herb has been of proven benefit in cases of epilepsy (particularly Grand Mal or major epilepsy) and research is still being carried out in some quarters to try and establish exactly which of it's active principles is beneficial to those who suffer from epileptiform attacks.

The roots of all the Elder species are extremely purgative and should be taken with caution.

Dosage: A tisane can be made from the flowerheads to Standard

Strength, but *be careful*, a sizeable number of species are poisonous. Be sure to identify the plant correctly.

Synonyms: Black Elder.

- **EYEBRIGHT** *Euphrasia officinalis*

Botanical information: The Eyebrights are a somewhat difficult group of plants, taxonomically speaking. There are over two hundred species, most of which are pseudo-parasitic annuals, all being members of the *Scrophulariaceae* family.

The Eyebrights can be found growing all over Europe, being indigenous to the Central and Eastern parts. *E. officinalis* flowers from May to October, and it is the flowerheads that should be collected then for medicinal purposes. July is the month during which the flowers are at their prime.

Therapeutic uses: The first choice in the treatment of opthalmic or eye disease. The active principles of Eyebright are still something of a mystery, but the plant is known to contain tannins, traces of mucilagens and some resins with antiseptic and anti-inflammatory properties. The plant also contains a variety of glycosides, but their exact nature and purpose are as yet undiscovered.

So enthusiastic was Culpepper about *E. officinalis* that he had this rather wry comment to make:

If the herb was as much used as it is neglected, it would half spoil the spectacle-makers' trade.

John Gerard had earlier remarked:

Eyebright stamped and laid upon the eyes, or the juice thereof mixed with White Wine, and dropped into the eyes, or the distilled water, taketh away the darknesse and dimnesse of the eyes, and cleareth the sight.

Dosage: The liquid extract of the flowers or a tisane should be used as eyedrops *pro re nata*.

Synonyms: Augentrost, Eufrasia.

- **FEVERFEW** *Crysanthemum parthenium*

Botanical information: Feverfew is of the *Compositae* family, and one of the *Pyrethrums*, a sub-genera of the *Tanacetums*. It grows wild in most parts of Europe, and is cultivated on a cottage basis for its medicinal value.

Therapeutic uses: The syllable 'few' in the name Feverfew derives from the Latin *fugo*, meaning 'put to flight'. This refers to the plants ability to remove pain, or metaphorically speaking, put it to flight. Feverfew is an excellent anodyne that seems particularly useful in cases of migraine and cramp that accompany the menses. It is also a mild sedative and euphoric, and is occasionally added to compound remedies for the relief of nervous tension.

In large doses it can sedate those who are suffering from nervous hysteria, but may produce some side-effects. However, in moderate doses the herb is completely safe.

Moderately high doses of Feverfew have been recommended (with some success) for the expulsion of the principle variety of roundworm *Ascaris lumbricoides,* but as the herb's vermicidal qualities are rather weak in comparison with those of other plant medicines, it seems best suited as an ingredient of a compound remedy.

Dosage: A tisane of standard strength should be made and taken twice a day, one ½ cupful at a time.

Synonyms: Featherfoil, Featherfew.

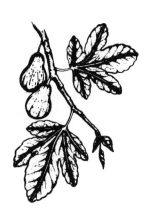

THE FIG (*Ficus carica*) is one of nature's natural antibiotics.

● **FIG** *Ficus carica*
Botanical information: A large pantropical genus of trees and shrubs
that are deciduous in cooler climates but evergreen in hotter regions.
There are approximately two-thousand species, including *F. carica*,
and they are of the *Moraceae* family.
Therapeutic uses: The Fig has always been highly regarded as a
medicinal herb, and it's use in the treatment of boils and other
localized inflammations has been well documented. The Bible itself
records how the Prophet Isaiah cured King Hezekiah, under
Jehovah's direction, of a boil that had apparently become
superinfected and was threatening his life:

> Isaiah proceeded to say: 'take a cake of pressed, dried figs and rub
> it upon the boil, that he may revive'.
>
> (2nd Kings 20:7)

American herbals particularly seem to emphasise the use of *F.
carica* in the treatment of boils. The herb gains a mention by Kadans,
and also by Ben Charles Harris in his *The Compleat Herbal*.
(Larchmont Books 1972)
The plant not only has remarkable antibiotic properties, but it also
acts as a disinfectant. A poultice of dried figs will considerably reduce
the foul stench given off by chronic ulcers on the legs if it is applied
directly to the wound.
Syrup of Figs is an excellent remedy for constipation, but has
fallen into disuse in recent times in many places with the advent of
modern laxatives.
Dosage: Syrup of Figs may be taken sparingly as required, or as
directed by your herbal practitioner.
Synonyms: Ficca.

● **FOXGLOVE** *Digitalis purpurea*
Botanical information: *D. purpurea*, a member of the *Scrophulariaceae*
family, is a biennial native of Western Europe, but is now also found
under cultivation in the U.S.A in New York, Washington, Utah and
Colorado.
The plant prefers soil with an acid bias, and favours woods and
copses in preference to exposed places. However, it is not
uncommon to find some varieties growing on the edge of moorland.

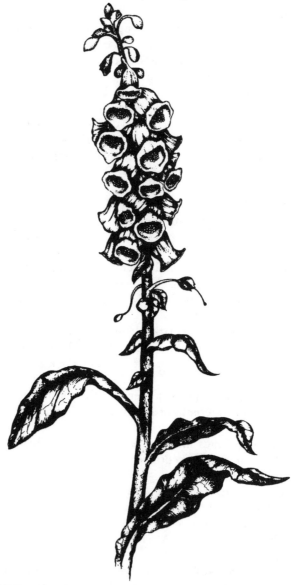

FOXGLOVE (*Digitalis purpurea*) is a famous remedy for heart-disease.

Therapeutic uses: The herb is rich in cardiac glycosides (*lanatosides*) and is therefore used to regulate and stimulate cardiac activity. Besides traces of saponins, the herb also contains powerful diuretic chemicals which have proved useful in the treatment of oedema or dropsy.

In recent years pharmaceutical manufacturers have tended to abandon *D. purpurea* in favour of its relative *D. lanata* which grows in Northern Europe and the Middle East. This herb produces the same therapeutic effects as *D. purpurea* but contains the active principles in greater quantities.

Dosage: Foxglove is deadly poisonous if taken in excess, and should never be ingested unless under medical supervision. Some countries have regulations prohibiting it's use except by trained physicians.

Synonyms: Fox Glue, Hanging Bells, Scrophula Herb.

● **GARLIC** *Allium sativum*

Botanical information: Garlic is a perennial plant of Oriental origin and a genus of the *Lilaceae*. It is widely cultivated in the Mediterranean area and throughout Asia for its medicinal properties. The bulbs (*Bulbus allii sativi*) are the parts used and they are harvested in July – September when the leaves turn yellow.

Therapeutic uses: The malodorous volatile oil in the garlic cloves has powerful medicinal properties. It contains organic sulphurs, several antibiotics and vitamins A, B complex and C. It also contains the rare trace element selenium and iron, phosphorous, potassium and calcium.

The antibiotic quality of Garlic has made it of use in the treatment of bronchial infections, intestinal fungi and blood disorders. The herb is also good for skin ailments but should *not* be applied externally in poultice form as it will severely irritate the dermis.

The plant also has a reputation as a vermifuge. Eating 2–3 garlic cloves a day should be all that is necessary, but in extreme cases it is reported that the Romanies, born masters of herbalism, will insert a garlic clove into the anus overnight. This may indeed work, but it should be remembered that the membrane lining the descending colon is easily irritated, and there are other herbal vermicides available that can be taken orally with little or no discomfort.

Garlic is also a reliable treatment for hypertension, but results do

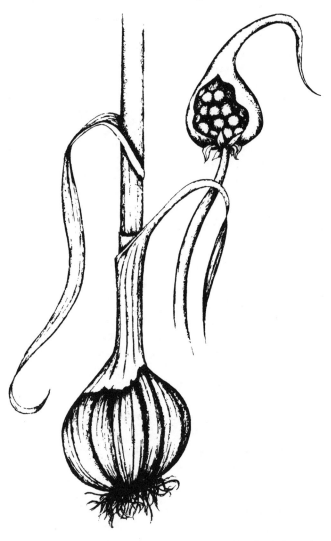

GARLIC (*Allium sativa*). Commonly known as the 'herbal antibiotic', Garlic is employed in the treatment of a wide variety of bacterial infections. It is also an aperient.

not come immediately. It may take up to four weeks before any significant change in the blood-pressure is noted.

Fuller commented:

> Not to speak of the murmuring Israelites, some avow it soveraigne for men and beasts in most maladies. Indeed a large book is written on it's virtues, which if held proportionate with truth, one should wonder any man should die, who hath garlic growing in his garden.

Dosage: The cloves may be eaten ad–lib, but not excessively.

Synonyms: Garlick, Gerlick.

- **GINSENG** *Panax quinquefolia*

Botanical information: *Panax* are a small genus of perennials native to the Orient and North America. There are around six species, all of them possessing the same chemical constituents in their roots to a greater or lesser extent.

Therapeutic uses: Perhaps no herb has excited so much interest in medical circles as Ginseng, and yet, strangely, it does not actually 'cure' any one ailment. Rather, it's virtues lie in it's tremendous power as a tonic and invigorator.

Korean chemico-botanists, amongst the most skilled in the world when it comes to plant-medicine research, have produced a root far superior to any other through a process of selective germination, and Korean Ginseng is now regarded as the finest in the world. Indeed, an old Oriental proverb says that if two men were to walk around the world non-stop, the one who looked untired and refreshed at the end of the journey would have a piece of Ginseng root hidden under his tongue!

Russian athletes are prescribed large amounts of Ginseng, because researchers in Moscow have shown that it not only improves stamina but also increases the efficiency with which blood is pumped to the muscles.

Ginseng cannot truly be classed as a sedative, but it is a good nervine. Ginseng tea seems to have a calming effect upon the system, and there is no better way to unwind after a tiring day than to sit down with a cup of Ginseng tea sweetened with honey.

Herbal practitioners in the U.S.A. have reported some success in treating anorexia with moderately high doses of Ginseng.

Dosage: Between 15–20 grains of the powdered herb can be taken three times a day, and a tisane made from the root can be drunk as desired.

Synonyms: Pannag, Man Root, Finger Root.

● **GOA** *Andira araroba*

Botanical information: The Goa tree is a member of the *Leguminosae*, the largest botanical family next to the grasses. It inhabits the forest areas of Brazil.

Therapeutic uses: Goa is an excellent vermifuge, and seems particularly effective against two of the three main varieties of tapeworm; *taenia mediocanellata*, normally found in infected beef, and *taenia solium*, the slightly less common variety normally found in infected pork. *A. araroba* is less successful it seems, against *dibothriocephalus latus*, normally found in infected fish.

The powdered and purified Araroba is also used in the treatment of skin diseases, and has even gained the sneaking admiration of some orthodox doctors because of it's effectiveness. The powder is mixed with a glycerine based ointment and applied to chronic ailments such as eczema, cystic acne and psoriasis.

Powdered Araroba (chemical name chrysarobine) can also be made into an antiseptic paint for use during surgical procedures.

Dosage: Only as prescribed by a qualified practitioner. Pure Goa or Araroba powder can severely irritate the eyes, nose and throat, and should never be applied directly to fungal infections of the inner thigh, as severe inflammation of the testicles may occur in males.

Synonyms: Bahia Powder, Ringworm Powder, Brazilian Dust.

● **GOLDEN ROD** *Solidago virga-aurea*

Botanical information: A genus of herbaceous perennials of the Compositae family, comprising of approximately one hundred and twenty-five species. Almost all the Goldenrods are found in the Americas, with the exception of several that can be found in Asia and an even smaller number that have adapted to the cooler climate of Europe.

Therapeutic uses: In the Americas *S. canadensis* is a widely used medicinal herb, and it possesses similar qualities to *S. virga-aurea*. The European species is not so potent, but is used almost exclusively

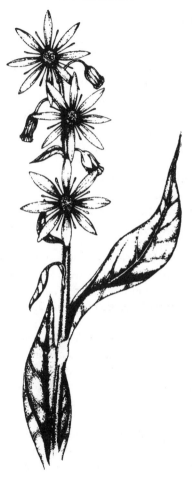

GOLDEN ROD (*Solidago virgaurea*) is used in the treatment of allergies.

here because of it's availability.

The herb has an agreeable effect upon the stomach and intestines, and as it is slightly aromatic it stimulates gastric activity.

The herb is also useful in cases of generalised oedema because it is diuretic and diaphoretic. Several oedemic patients have also noticed a beneficial side effect, namely the catabolism or breaking down of

stones in the urinary tract. Indeed, the Amerindians have long used
S. canadensis as a treatment for urinary calculi.

Orthodox researchers have shown some interest in Golden Rod as
a treatment for hay-fever. The plant contains much pollen, normally
an allergen, and yet hay-fever sufferers do not seem to be affected
when in close proximity to the plant. Herbal and homoeopathic
preparations of Golden Rod have been used successfully in the
treatment of hay-fever and other allergies.

Dosage: An infusion of Standard Strength should be taken four times
a day, a ½ cupful at one time.

Synonyms: Aaron's Rod, Woundwort, Goldenrods.

● **GROUNDSEL**   *Senecio vulgaris*

Botanical information: The *Senecio* genus is one of the largest
amongst the flowering plants and accounts for more than 1,500
species within the *Compositae* family.

S. *vulgaris* grows on wasteland and arable soil, and thrives near
coastal areas and on beaches. It flowers for most of the year.

Therapeutic uses: Groundsel is not the most popular, or the most
attractive, of medicinal herbs, but it has an impressive history as a
medicine.

The Greek physician Dioscorides (Pedanius) (c. 40A.D.–90A.D.)
recommended Groundsel in his classic work *De Materia Medica,* and
the two fathers of modern English herbalism, Gerard and
Culpeper, both advocated it's use. Gerard said that 'the leaves of
Groundsel boiled in wine or water, and drunke, healed the paine and
ach of the stomacke that proceeds choler.'

Modern herbals still recommend Groundsel as a remedy for
biliousness, and it is also used as a soothing refrigerant for teething
babies – another practice dating back to the Middle Ages.

As the alkaloids within the plant are known to inhibit cell division
some researchers are hopeful that it may some day be possible to
isolate the active principles and use them to slow down or arrest the
growth of malignant tumours, but such research is still in it's
infancy.

Dosage: Small doses of S. *vulgaris* are harmless, but is unwise to state
dosages here as there is considerable evidence to suggest that
excessive use, even over short periods, may cause cirrhosis of the

liver. I would therefore recommend that the herb only be taken under supervision.

Synonyms: Grounsel, Grundsle.

● **GUARANA** *Paullinia cupara*

Botanical information: A Brazilian plant of the *Sapindaceae* family that has many medical and commercial uses.

Therapeutic uses: The roasted seeds of the plant are ground and then mixed into paste which is cut into strips and dried. The herb is rich in caffeine, and has understandably become a popular stimulant amongst the natives. At least one soft drinks manufacturer is now marketing a Guarana-flavoured beverage.

The caffeine content makes the herb moderately useful in relieving some kinds of headache, and because it has diuretic properties it has also been used in the treatment of urinary infections by Brazilian herbalists.

Dosage: Between 10–50 grains of the powdered root, as directed.

Synonyms: Guarano, Brazilian Cocoa, Uabano, Wachite, Uaranazeiro.

● **HEARTSEASE** *Viola tricolor*

Botanic information: The *Violas* are a large genus of perennials that are widely distributed throughout the temperate zones. They are native to Europe, but naturalized in North America. Most of the cultivated Pansies are derived from *Viola tricolor,* which flowers during Spring and Summer.

Therapeutic uses: *V. tricolor* contains saponins, salicylic acid compounds and flavones, and is used chiefly in the treatment of blood disorders, but it's actions on the circulatory system are not precisely known. It has detergent and antiseptic qualities which may assist the removal of antigens (foreign bodies) from the blood stream. It is also mildly diuretic.

V. tricolor has also been used in the treatment of epileptic disorders (both grand and petit mal) and similar ailments. It has a depressant effect upon the nervous system, and also dilates the bronchi, which helps relieve the symptoms of asthma.

Dosage: As prescribed by a practitioner. *V. tricolor* may effect cardiac action if taken in excess.

Synonyms: Love In Idleness, Three Hooded Faces, Johnny-Jump-

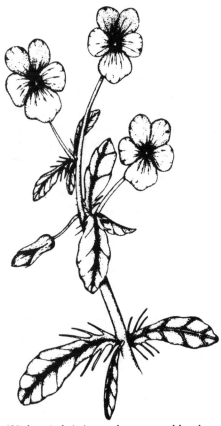

HEARTSEASE (*Viola tricolor*) is used to treat blood and circulatory disorders.

Up, Johnny-Jump-Me-Up, Johnny-Jump-Up-Me, Field Pansy, European Wild Pansy.

● **HEMLOCK**   *Conicum maculatum*

Botanical information: A biennial or perennial herb of the *Umbelliferae,* flowering in June or July. It grows throughout temperate Europe and Eurasia, and also to a smaller extent in the U.S.A., Australia and New Zealand.

Therapeutic uses: When the Greek philosopher Socrates constantly ridiculed the conventional wisdom of his religious contemporaries, he eventually ended up in court, not surprisingly, on a charge of 'impiety and the corruption of our youth'. Having been found guilty, he was sentenced to death in the year 402 B.C., and the sentence was carried out two years later. The mode of execution was simple. Socrates would drink a brew made from Hemlock, one of the worst poisons in the plant kingdom. Death came by a slow, progressive failure of the respiratory system.

And yet Hemlock has some virtues. If taken in small amounts it can relieve the symptoms of epilepsy, chorea, nervous hysteria and similar afflictions, as it is a sedative and anodyne.

It's depressant activity relieves bronchial spasms, and it has been used with some success on children suffering from whooping-cough.

Dosage: None can be safely recommended for the lay herbalist. NEVER attempt to use *C. maculatum* or it's relative species *Cicuta maculatum* (Water Hemlock) as a medicine unless well qualified to do so.

Synonyms: Poison Hemlock, Parsley Poison, Poison Parsley.

● **HENNA** *Lawsonia alba*
Botanical information: Henna is the dye extracted from the herb *L. alba* of the *Lythraceae* family. It has been cultivated in the tropics since ancient times and is now grown successfully in various parts of the Americas.

Therapeutic uses: The dye is normally used to colour the hair, or, in the case of some African tribes, certain parts of the body. Medicinally speaking, the history of Henna has been most thoroughly documented in India, where physicians have long placed great stock on it's curative properties and prescribed it not only for minor ailments such as migraine and brittle nails, but also for venereal disease, leprosy, smallpox and gangrene.

The leaves are rich in calcium oxalate.

Dosage: As directed.

Synonyms: Henne, Alhenne, Alhenna, Hennha.

● **HONEYSUCKLE** *Lonicera caprifolium*
Botanical information: A large genus of Caprifoliaceous shrub found throughout the Northern Hemisphere and the Americas, (particularly Mexico). *L. caprifolium* grows in abundance in both the U.K. and west Asia, and flowers during the month of June.

Therapeutic uses: Honeysuckle was one of the many medicinal herbs that John Gerard grew in his private garden, and he recommended that the 'floures, be steeped in oile, and set in the Sun, are good to annoint the body that is benummed, and growne very cold'.

Miller reiterates this in his herbal, where he says; 'The oil, made by Infusion of the Flowers, is accounted healing and warming, and good for the Cramp and the Convulsions of the Nerves.'

An oil made from the flowers of the Honeysuckle and gently heated is a fine way to restore the circulation to the extremities that have been numbed by the cold. The plant has vasodilative properties that cause an increase in blood flow to the dermis, and these active principles are readily absorbed by the skin with the oil.

In times past the decoction of the flowerheads was added to a syrup and used as a cough linctus. A tisane is also said to be useful in cases of asthma.

Lonicera villosa or American Honeysuckle is used in the U.S.A and Canada as a kidney stimulant.

Dosage: A tisane can be made to standard strength and taken three teaspoonfuls at a time, four times a day. Tisanes are best made from the leaves of the plant.

Synonyms: Dutch Honeysuckle, Woodbine, Wood-Bind, Honey Suckle.

- **HOPS** *Humulus lupulus*

Botanical information: A small genus of annual or perennial shrubs of the *Moraceae* family, comprising of just two species.

H. lupulus is widely cultivated for it's strobiles or catkins which contain *lupulin resins*. During the brewing of beer, lupulin resins are converted chemically to *iso-humulones,* the bitter principle which gives beer it's distinctive bitter flavour as opposed to ale, which does not contain hops.

Therapeutic uses: A by-product of hops used in the brewing process is the chemical *lupuline,* an effective sedative that has proved useful in cases of insomnia. A tisane taken just before one retires to bed is a night-assured means of gaining a good night's sleep. Unlike some mineral based sedatives and tranquilizers, *H. lupulus* has no untoward side effects, and the user will awake the following morning feeling refreshed.

Hop tea is also useful in cases of atonic or debilitative dyspepsia, in

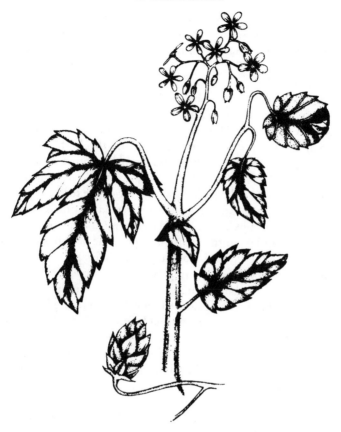

THE COMMON HOP (*Humulus lupulus*) is an effective sedative.

which the muscle-tone of the stomach wall is weakened due to illness or old age.

Dosage: Tisane of Standard Strength.

Synonyms: Hoppe.

- **HORE-HOUND** *Marrubium vulgare*
Botanical information: A genus of perennials of the *Labiatae* family, *Marrubium* is native to Eurasia and the Mediterranean area, but now naturalized in South and Central Europe, North America and the U.K.

The plant is cultivated in many areas of the British Isles, and its aromatic principles are used in confections and in the making of liqueurs. The plant is not often found growing wild, but if you do come across it, it will likely be in a sunny exposure with moist, nutrient-rich soil.

Therapeutic uses: Of all the herbs used in the treatment of pulmonary and bronchial disorders, there is no finer pectoral and expectorant than Hore-Hound. It contains a unique bitter principle (*marrubin*) which is directly responsible for the herb's ability to remove mucous from the lungs and bronchi, and it is this same chemical that acts as an appetite stimulant: most beneficial in influenza cases where the patient has lost the desire to eat.

Horehound is also known to have several uses in the fields of gynaecology and obstetrics. Besides having a reputation as an alterative in disorders of the menstrual cycle, the herb has also been used to facilitate the expulsion of the placenta after parturition. This is achieved by taking a strong tisane or decoction of the herb immediately after the birth, but it must be stated at this point that the use of *M. vulgare* in this regard has not been subjected to proper scrutiny, and ANY herb taken during labour (or indeed at any time during gestation) should only be done so under strict supervision.

Several old herbals recommend Hore-Hound for 'bringing down the flow' and to 'start the bleedings', indicating the the herb is beneficial in cases of amenorrhoea.

Dosage: A tisane of Standard Strength.

Synonyms: Hoarhound, Hoar-Hound, Horehound, White Horehound, Marvel, Marrubium.

● **HORSETAIL** *Equisetum arvense*

Botanical information: The *Equisetum* or Horsetail genus is the only group of the *Sphenophytina*, an order of vascular plants. There are sixteen known species and eighteen hybrids. Botanically speaking, they fall somewhere between the ferns and the clubmosses.

Of the sixteen known species, eleven can be found in the British Isles, and they grow most prolifically in the North East and North West of England, and the lowland areas of Scotland.

Like all Horsetails, *E. arvense* does not flower, but produces spore-sacs which are visible from March to September.

Therapeutic uses: The Horsetails have not been investigated as well as most other genera for their medicinal virtues, and considerable confusion still exists over their precise effects on the human physiology.

It has been established that the plant contains silicic acid, saponins, alkaloids and a poisonous substance called thiaminase which causes symptoms of toxicity in both humans and animals.

Almost all the older herbals recommend *E. arvense* as a styptic for arresting the flow of blood from external wounds, and whilst it does seem to have some value in this regard its use in preventing or arresting internal bleeding is dubious.

It is still popular in some parts to prescribe *E. arvense* as a diuretic, but this seems illogical when other, less toxic, herbs can be used just as efficiently. Thiaminase poisoning causes a deficiency of vitamin B1 (Hypovitaminosis B1) and may also cause permanent liver damage.

Dosage: Until further research establishes a safe dosage for use in home medication, take as directed by your practitioner.

Synonyms: Shave Grass, Pewterwort, Bottlebrush, Bottle Brush, Dutch Rushes, Hollander Rush Grass.

● **HOUSELEEK** *Sempervivum tectorum*

Botanical information: The forty different species of Houseleek are members of the *Crassulaceae* family. They are a common garden plant in Europe and also grow wild in Asia and North Africa.

The plant has an almost legendary ability to survive long periods of time without water. One popular story, no doubt somewhat exaggerated, concerns the botanist who tried for eighteen months, without success, to dry the plant for addition to his collection of wild flowers. Eventually, the story goes, he gave up and returned the plant to its original location where it flourished as if it had never been disturbed!

Therapeutic uses: In ancient times the plant was used by the Anglo-Saxons to treat skin ulcers and infected battle wounds. Today, the leaves are sliced or crushed and applied in poultice form to burns, warts, insect bites, corns, acneous lesions and other skin inflammations or growths.

Dosage: Apply externally in poultice form.

Synonyms: Common Houseleek, Thor's Beard, Stonecrop.

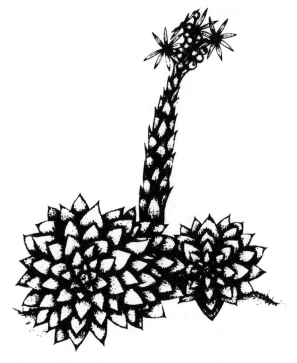

HOUSELEEK (*Sempervivum tectorum*) is a herbal remedy for bruises and external wounds.

● **ICELAND MOSS**   *Cetraria islandica*
Botanical information: A genus of lichen that inhabits the Arctic areas, and is used as a foodstuff by deer and caribou. The forty species of *Cetraria* belong to the *Parmeliaceae* family.
Therapeutic uses: As well as cattle fodder, *C. islandica* has also been used as a nutritious foodstuff by Icelanders, Norwegians, Laplanders and the Canadian Indians.

It is used almost exclusively in the treatment of chest and bronchial ailments, and is an excellent demulcent. It is rich in mucilagens and is added to several commercial cough remedies.

The herb also has a mildly beneficial effect on the digestive organs, particularly the stomach and small intestine. Indeed, an old Danish proverb says that if a person swallows a handful of Iceland Moss after

ˈtaking poison, then no harm will come to him. Of course this is entirely fallacious, but it illustrates the fact that the herb *does* have a soothing effect upon the delicate mucous membranes of the digestive tract. Its therapeutic action in this regard is due almost entirely to the presence of a glutinous, starchy mucilagen called *lichenine* which forms a protective barrier around inflamed tissue.

Dosage: A weak tisane ½ oz of the dried herb should be added to 1 pint of water.

Synonyms: Iceland lichen, Islandiches Moos, Consumption Moss.

● **JALAP** *Ipomoea purga*

Botanical information: Jalap is the resin collected from the tubers of *I. purga,* a climbing plant that inhabits the Mexican Andes and parts of Peru. The herb is of the *Convolvulaceae* family.

Therapeutic uses: The resin from the root is a powerful purgative and is used to facilitate bowel evacuation in the most drastic cases of constipation and intestinal torpor.

The laxative action of the herb is so strong that it is normally used in compound remedies rather than as a simple. It may be combined with *Zingiber officinale* (Ginger), *Glycyrrhiza glabra* (Licorice), *Lewisia rediviva* (Spathum) or some other digestive stimulant, and used as an aperient or purgative depending on the amount of I. purga added to the mixture.

The herb also has a mild anodyne/antispasmodic quality, and some herbals (Milthorpe's and Smith's) have remarked on its usefulness in relieving spasms in the gut.

Dosage: 5–10 grains of the powdered herb. Due to its drastic cathartic action, only 1–2 grains of the herb should be taken initially, and the full dosage several hours later under supervision.

Synonyms: Purge Root.

● **JAMBUL** *Eugenia jambolana*

Botanical information: *Eugenia,* a large, warm-temperate genus of evergreens, contains a number of trees and shrubs with edible fruits/seeds and sundry medicinal virtues. Many species are found almost exclusively in South America, unlike *E. jambolana* which also thrives in India and Australia.

Therapeutic uses: The seeds of Jambul are widely reputed to be useful in cases of sugar diabetes. Tests have shown that even small dosages, preceded by an initial dose of fifteen grains, will rapidly reduce blood and urine sugar levels. A maintainance dose of 3–5 grains is reputed to keep the blood sugar level in control.

Why, then, is Jalap not used more widely, and heralded as the answer to diabetes? Quite simply, because it only seems to work with a frustratingly small percentage of diabetics, and the orthodox medical fraternity have not, to my knowledge, carried ot a full investigation into its chemico-therapeutic qualities.

Dosage: An initial dosage of fiteen grains for an adult, and a maintainance dose as directed by a physician or health practitioner.

WARNING: The Department of Health do NOT recommend that any form of diabetes be treated with self-medication.

Synonyms: Java Plum, Jambu, Rose Apple Thorn.

● **JEWEL WEED** *Impatiens biflora*

Botanical information: *Impatiens*, a genus of annuals and perennials with a moderately wide distribution, can be found in Africa, the Americas, Eurasia and in several other mountainous climes around the world. There are over six-hundred species, and they belong to the *Balsamaceae* family.

Therapeutic uses: *I. biflora* has a wide variety of medicinal uses. It is an aperient, being useful in cases of mild constipation, and also stimulates liver activity. It has thus been used as an adjunctive treatment for jaundice and some hepatic-related opthalmic conditions.

The comminuted herb can be added to a hydrogenated fat and used as an external treatment for hemorrhoids and other varicose conditions. It also has parasiticidal qualities, and can be used to treat certain skin infections. The herb contains several glycosides that are effective in treating two types of ringworm: *Tinea tonsurans* and *Tinea sycosis*. The herb is also effecive against *Tinea circinata*, but not to the same degree. However, *T. circinata* is a particularly intractable form of the disease.

I. biflora has diuretic qualities and has been used in the treatment of dropsy.

Dosage: A tisane can be made to Standard Strength and taken three times a day, one fl. oz. at a time. The tisane can also be used as an antiseptic skin wash.

Synonyms: Pale Touch-Me-Not, Touch-Me-Not, Wild Celandine,

Spotted Touch-Me-Not, Speckled Jewels, Balsam Weed, Wild Balsam, Balsam A' Florae.

● **JOHN'S BREAD** *Ceratonia siliqua*

Botanical information: A species of the *Leguminosae* family that has been the subject of extensive cultivation in the Mediterranean area and in the Middle East. The large, sweet-tasting pods are extremely nutritious and were a common sight in British confectionery shops until the late 1950's. They are still available in many health-food stores and at some surgical suppliers.

The plant is now often called Carob, and is used as a chocolate substitute. It is also confused with several other species, most commonly, *Parkia filicoidea* (West African Locust Bean), *Robinia pseudoacacia* (Black Locust), *Hymenaea courbaril* (Locust Tree) and *Gleditsia triacanthos* (Locust Honey Tree). Amateur herbalists also often confuse the plant with *Hypericum perforatum* (St. John's Wort).

There has long been speculation (since at least 300 A.D.) that the herb was used by John the Baptizer to sustain him in the wilderness, but this is not attested to by the Bible account (Matthew 3:4) which most definitely says that he ate 'locusts', a clean animal food for the Jews under the Mosaic Law. (Locust is a common name for John's Bread.)

Therapeutic uses: The medicinal use of *C.siliqua* is rather obscure. Besides being extremely nutritious, it also is said to have a beneficial effect upon the larynx, relaxing and toning the vocal chords, and also improve breathing. The comminuted pod also has styptic properties, and will arrest bleeding if it is dusted over a wound.

Dosage: The pods may be eaten *ad lib* but in moderation.

Synonyms: Carob, Caroba, St. John's Bread, Locust.

● **JUNIPER** *Juniperus communis*

Botanical information: The Junipers are a genus of evergreens popular in the Northern Hemisphere. There are over seventy species of Juniper, all of them having some nutritional, medicinal or commercial use. *J. communis* is the most popular, and the one that concerns us specifically.

Therapeutic uses: Oil of Juniper is used to flavour Gin, and not only does it give the spirit its characteristic flavour, but it also seems to imbue it with a depressant effect slightly more than that caused by

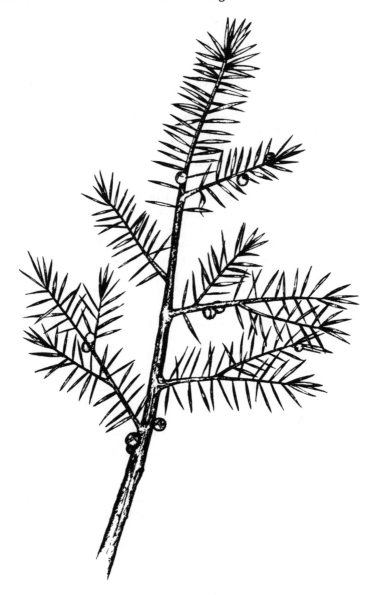

COMMON JUNIPER (*Juniperus communis*) is an effective sedative.

the alcohol itself. This gives some credence to the old wives' tale that 'Gin makes you feel depressed'.

The herb was also used as a sedative in ancient times, being mentioned in Greek and Arabic herbals.

Presently, the herb is used as a diuretic and seems to be particularly useful in the treatment of cystitis.

Dosage: 10 grains of the solid extract.

Synonyms: Horse Savin.

● **KOLA** *Cola nitida*

Botanical information: *C. nitida* is the main cultivated species of Kola, and thrives in the rain forests of South and West Africa, Sierra Leone and other countries. The tree is cultivated for its 'nuts' which are stimulants. Kola production is now estimated to be over 180,000 tonnes per year, and Nigeria is the greatest producer.

Therapeutic uses: The unique, stimulating properties of Kola are explained by its chemical make-up. One nut contains up to 2% caffeine, and also *theobromine* and *colanin*: all stimulants. The herb is completely safe in small doses, and can be a tremendous pick-me-up in cases of fatigue. However, the use of artificial stimulants is contraindicated unless required for a sound medical reason. Caffeine is both physically and psychologically addictive.

The caffeine content also makes the herb a useful diuretic, and it is an excellent remedy for diarrhoea because of its astringency.

Kola can be used as a cardiac stimulant, but large doses will produce arrythmia and its use should be monitored carefully.

Dosage: 28 grains of the powdered herb in twenty four hours should be sufficient.

Synonyms: Kola Nut, Cola Nut, Kolla Nut.

● **LADY'S MANTLE** *Alchemilla vulgaris*

Botanical information: A large genus of American, European and Asian perennials that grow at montane elevations. Of the three-hundred and fifty species, only *A. vulgaris* has been of any real therapeutic benefit. The Lady's Mantles belong to the *Rosaceae* family.

Therapeutic uses: Used as a styptic for the treatment of both internal and external bleeding. The early herbals recommend it for the treatment of menorrhagia, but it is best taken as part of a compound remedy as opposed to a simple.

The real advantage of the herb lies in its extremely powerful action, which, if the herb is taken in the correct dosages, will produce no untoward side-effects. The active constituent in the herb seems to be its high content of tannins. These cause the astringent action which arrests bleeding.

Despite the herb's styptic action, it must be remembered that arresting any form of haemorrhage is simply a palliative measure that does not remove the cause of the problem. Wounds that take unusually long to stop bleeding, or bleeding from the eyes, nose, throat, mouth or anus (or in the sexually mature bleeding from the sexual organs), should receive professional attention.

The comminuted herb is said to produce an antiseptic action when mixed with *Polygonum bistorta* (Snakeweed).

Dosage: Tisane of Standard Strength.

Synonyms: Lion's Foot.

● **LEMON**   *Citrus Limonia*

Botanical information: The lemon is of Indian origin but is now naturalized in many areas of the world with a warm climate. It is the citrus fruit of premier importance to the food industry, and accounts for 10% of all citrus fruits grown.

Therapeutic uses: Lemon is an excellent febrifuge and is universally acknowledged as a good home remedy for colds and influenza. It possesses bactericidal qualities that can be enhanced by the action of some other 'natural antibiotics' such as *Eucalyptus globulus* (Eucalyptus) and honey. It is added to the former as a treatment for throat infections and to the latter as an antibiotic febrifuge in cases of influenza.

The peel or rind of the lemon has been used pharmaceutically and is often used as a flavouring agent in cakes. However, it is likely to cause nausea if taken in excess.

An old Bulgarian folk-remedy for cuts suggests painting lemon juice onto cuts to promote quick healing, but this can be a painful procedure due to the citric acid content!

Dosage: Ad lib.

Synonyms: Limon, Limone, Lemone.

● **LICORICE**   *Glycyrrhiza glabra*

Botanical information: A woody perennial of the *Papilionaceae* family that grows in the Mediterranean area, Russia and India. The

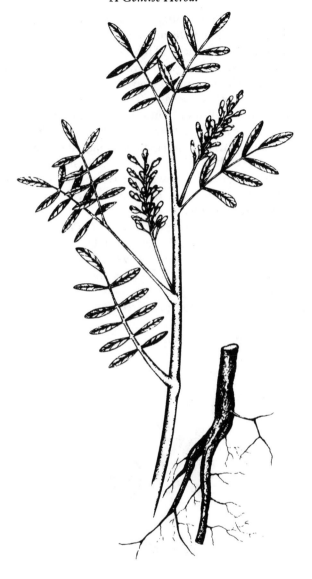

LICORICE (*Glycyrrhiza glabra*) is added to many commercial drugs for the treatment of stomach ulcers.

herb is also cultivated on a cottage basis in some areas of the U.K., particularly Yorkshire and Nottinghamshire.

Therapeutic uses: Unlike many of the lesser known medicinal herbs, the therapeutic actions of *G. glabra* have been well researched.

The most useful ingredient is a sapo-glycoside called *glycyrrhizin* – fifty times as sweet as sucrose. This, combined with another flavonoid glycoside called liquiritosidin (liquiritoside) has a healing action on the stomach. The herb is used by many pharmaceutical companies (particularly in Holland) as an ingredient in treatments for stomach ulcers, although its efficacy has been disputed by some researchers. Most herbalists, however, have no such doubts, and still prescribe a tisane made from the comminuted roots for ulcers, gastritis and related disorders.

Another use of *G. glabra* is in the treatment of bronchitis and sore throats. It is an expectorant and suppressant. Holt says: 'It is the most calming of all the herbs for taking away the soreness in the throat.'

Licorice also happens to be a laxative and should be used with some discretion.

Dosage: 10 to 30 grains of the powdered root, or the whole root can be chewed *ad lib*.

Synonyms: Liquorice, Licorish.

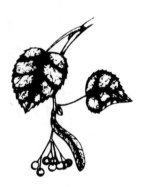

LIME (*Citrus medica*) is antiseptic and astringent.

● **LIME FLOWER**   *Tilea europea*

Botanical information: A deciduous ornamental tree that grows in Europe and also in large quantities in the Eastern states of North America.

Therapeutic uses: Some confusion exists as to which of *T. europea's* medicinal qualities is the most beneficial. Some authorities place great emphasis on its use as a nervine, and it is true that the herb rivals Chamomile in some parts of Germany as a treatment for PMT (pre-menstrual tension). Larger doses have also been used with varying degrees of success in the treatment of convulsions and hysteria.

Conversely, the herb is equally as popular in some parts of the world because of its anti-inflammatory properties, and the Basques, by way of example, recommend it for the treatment of stomach ulcers.

The herb also contains saponins and mucilagens, and has a mild expectorant action. It can be used in cases of bronchitis and similar ailments.

Dosage: A tisane of Standard Strength to be taken *pro re nata.*

Synonyms: Lindenflower, Linden, Lindleflower.

● **LUNGWORT**   *Lobaria pulmonaceae*

Botanical information: A lichen that grows in damp climates and is usually found in close proximity to one of two trees; *Fraxinus excelsior* (Ash) and *Fagus sylvatica* (Beech). Found in many temperate climates.

Therapeutic uses: *L. pulmonaceae* is rich in acid bitters which have two primary effects upon the constitution. Firstly, they promote the production and secretion of digestive enzymes throughout the entire digestive tract, and secondly, they increase the efficiency with which the digestive processes work by encouraging the breakdown of proteins into peptides in the stomach.

The herb has also been used in cases of pulmonary tuberculosis, but its action is weaker in this regard than that of *Cetraria islandica* (Iceland Moss).

Dosage: Tisane of Standard Strength.

Synonyms: Oak Lungs,Lungmoss, False Iceland Moss.

● **MANNA**   *Fraxinus ornus*

Botanical infromation: The common name Manna is a misleading one, for it can be applied to the sticky exudate from any herb or tree in the plant kingdom. In this case, the name refers to *F. ornus*, the Manna Ash which grows throughout Europe but chiefly in Italy.

Therapeutic uses: A mild aperient that is used to treat constipation in children and expectant mothers. It is rich in carbohydrates and other nutrients, and may be added to Slippery Elm and Agar-Agar, also nutritious foodstuffs, as a sweetener.

Dosage: 1 teaspoonful as needed in milk; or if taken during pregnancy, as directed by your physician. Laxatives should NOT be taken during pregnancy unless under medical supervision.

Synonyms: Sweet Manna, Flake Manna, Manna Ash.

● **MARSHMALLOW** *Althaea officinalis*

Botanical information: A perennial herb of the *Malvaceae* family that grows throughout Europe and favours a marshy, acid-based soil. In the U.K. it can be found mainly in coastal areas, but is rare in some parts of the North of Scotland. The herb flowers from August to September, but it is the root and leaves that are used for medicinal purposes.

Therapeutic uses: The herb is useful in the treatment of coughs, but as its action is somewhat weak most herbals that deal with its properties at any length recommend that it is added to a compound and not prescribed on its own.

The herb has long been recommended as a cure for inflammation of the bladder, urethra and ureters, but its efficacy has been disputed by some experts (Flück and Sullivan). The chief criticism often made is that *A. officinalis* contains no really powerful antibiotic substances. However, as a tisane made from the plant is known to relax the muscular wall of the bladder significantly, it may be that pockets of stale urine are emptied and the number of bacteria in the bladder thereby reduced.

Marshmallow tea may be taken for digestive disorders as it is an emolient. This is by far the most popular use to which the plant is put in the U.K.

Dosage: A tisane of Standard Strength may be take *ad lib*.

Synonyms: Mallards, Schloss, Malvavisco, Kitmi, Bismalva.

● **MESCALE** *Lopophora lewinii*

Botanical information: The *Lopophora*, a genus of dwarf cactii, consist of just two species; *L. lewinii (L. williamsii) and L. diffusa. L.*

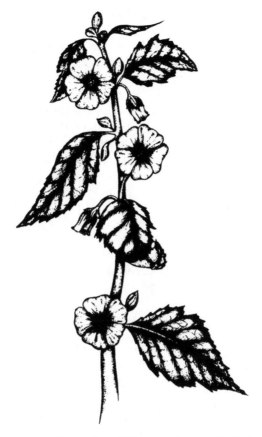

MARSHMALLOW (*Althaea officinalis*) is a popular remedy for bronchitis.

lewinii has an unparalleled place in the plant culture of the Americas. It is the 'sacred cactus' of the Mexican people and has been used for millenia as a hallucinogenic drug in pagan rituals.

   L. diffusa, which is restricted to Central Mexico, grows between Sierra Madre Occidental and Sierra Oriental. The genus is part of the *Cactaceae* family.

Therapeutic uses: The fruit of the plant contains the active principles, a variety of narcotic alkaloids, the most powerful of which is mescaline.

In anything over very small doses the fruits, sometimes called 'magic mushrooms' will produce a hallucinogenic effect similar to L.S.D. In fact, the plant was banned in most areas of the U.S.A. during the 1960s when the taking of narcotic drugs such as L.S.D. reached frightening proportions.

In larger amounts the herb produces symptoms of toxicity including vomiting, stupor, breathing difficulties etc, and therapeutic doses must be worked out very carefully. If the herb is prescribed correctly it can be of some benefit in cases of asthma and angina. The Mexican Indians who use the plant on a regular basis may suffer the various and inevitable symptoms of drug abuse, but it must also be said that they have a remarkably low incidence of cardio-vascular disease. Of course, there are a variety of possible explanations for this, but one strong possibility is that the alkaloids in Mescale reduce the coronary failure rate because they act as vasodilators.

Dosage: None can be safely recommended.

Synonyms: Muscal Buttons, Mescal Buttons, Pelote, Mescala, Magic Mushroom, Dream Cactus.

● **MISTLETOE**   *Viscum album*

Botanical information: The Mistletoes, including *V. album*, are members of the *Loranthaceae* family. They are parasites (actually, semi-parasitic) that seed in the host plant (fruit trees and occasionally the Horse Chestnut) and drain fluid in it for sustenance.

V. album is the most important, medicinally speaking, of the 1,300 species.

Therapeutic uses: Mistletoe may not be the greatest of medicinal herbs but it certainly ranks as one of the most controversial. The drug Iscador, imported into the U.K. by the Waleda company, is widely believed to be an anti-cancer agent and contains extract of Mistletoe. Although the company themselves make no 'cancer cure' claims for Iscador, some G.P.s use it and claim a reasonably high success rate. Others however, are completely sceptical.

The D.H.S.S. occasionally receive petitions from various medical bodies with an axe to grind who would like to see the sale of Mistletoe-based drugs restricted. Sometimes, their criticisms go overboard. One prominent doctor recently criticized a herbal O.T.C. remedy which, he said, contained Mistletoe. Subsequent checks with the manufacturer revealed that the product contained no

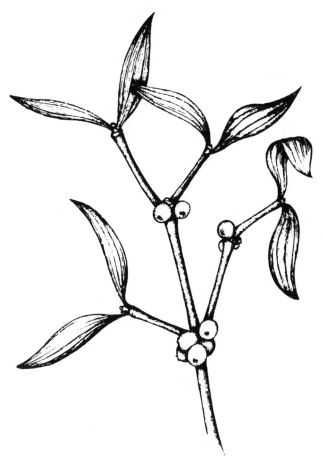

MISTLETOE (*Viscum album*). Used in the treatment of hypertension and cardiac diseases. Some attempts have also been made to treat inoperable forms of cancer with the herb.

Mistletoe at all, and more than one irate herbalist penned a response to the criticisms to the national press in a mood of righteous indignation.

So then, what exactly *is* Mistletoe good for? Gerard expounded on its beauty, but attributed little to it in the way of medicinal virtues.

And Culpeper, in his herbal, really added little to what Gerard had already said. However, the plant has achieved a tremendous reputation not only as an anticarcinogenic but also as an antispasmodic, sedative and tonic. It is particularly recommended in cases of epilepsy.

The herb is also rich in choline which can be employed in the treatment of hypertension or high blood pressure, and in the U.S.A it is used as an emolient and remedy for skin ailments. Some pharmaceutical companies still use it today.

It is in the treatment of cancer however, that the herb is the subject of greatest controversy. Some authorities (Flück) give a guarded credence to its efficacy, whilst others, like Dr. David Phillipson of London University's Pharmacognosy Department, seem mainly concerned over its toxicity.

Dosage: Only to be taken under supervision as the plant contains large amounts of viscotoxins.

Synonyms: Misselto, Misseltoe.

- **MOUNTAIN OREGON GRAPE** *Berberis aquifolium*

Botanical information: *The Barberries or Berberii* are members of the *Berberidaceae* family and there are over four-hundred and fifty species. The Mountain Oregon Grape *(B. aquifolium)* grows in California, several other areas of the U.S.A. and in British Columbia.

Therapeutic uses: *B. aquifolium* is a sadly underestimated herb that has not received proper scientific investigation. The bark has been used as a general tonic and stimulant to the digestive system, and it improves the absorbtion of nutrients in the gut.

In the United States the herb has gained a reputation as a treatment for infectious diseases such as typhoid and tuberculosis (in its early stages). It is also employed in cases of bilitis because of its anti-inflammatory properties and its mild anodyne content.

Kadans suggests that it may be useful in cases of syphilis, but Harris makes no mention of it in his *Compleat Herbal*.

Dosage: 10–30 drops of the liquid extract. A preserve may be made from the fruits and eaten *ad lib*. A related species *(B. vulgaris)* may be poisonous.

Synonyms: Sourberry, Oregon Grape, Berberry, Holly-Leaved

Berberry, Berberis, Oregon Berberina, Oregon Grape Root, Berberitze.

- **NUX-VOMICA** *Strychnos nux-vomica*

Botanical information: A widespread and diversified tropical and sub-tropical genus, the species of which are characterized by the fact that they call contain the poisonous alkaloid strychnine in their fruits or seeds.

S. *nux-vomica* is a tree that grows commonly in Burma, India and Sri Lanka, and also to a lesser extent in China and Australia. The fruit seeds contain the two most utilized active principles, the aforementioned *strychnine* and another, *brucine*.

Therapeutic uses: The seeds are therapeutic in very small amounts. They have been recommended for such divrse conditions as neuralgia, dyspepsia, impotence and constipation. It seems likely that the therapeutic value of the plant has been greatly exaggerated, and it is interesting to note that it gains but a scant mention, if at all, amongst any of the ancient herbals. Indeed, most ancient authorities held *Nux Vomica* in contempt, and its only real value is probably as a nervine and sedative.

Dosage: Extremely poisonous: not to be taken.

Synonyms: Quakers Buttons, Poison Nut.

- **OLIVE** *Olea europaea*

Botanical information: The olive is one of the most documented plants in history. It is mentioned repeatedly in the Bible, and the trees have the distinction of being one of the longest surviving species in the plant kindom. There are olive trees still flourishing today in Europe and the Middle East that were in existence during the time of Christ. They commonly grow to be 1,500 years old. They are of the family *Oleaceae*.

Therapeutic uses: Used primarily in the treatment of bowel diseases. It is an excellent laxative for children, but dosage should be monitored carefully.

O. *europaea* is also an antispasmodic and will relieve the pain of intestinal colic. It has been recommended as a vermifuge, but may need to be taken over a prolonged period to be successful.

Externally the herb oil can be applied to all manner of burns, scalds, sores and skin inflammation. Small eczemous patches of dry skin often respond well if they are coated frequently with olive oil, particularly those on the hands.

Dosage: Internally, one teaspoonful as required. Externally the oil may be applied *ad lib*.

Synonyms: Lucca.

● **ONION**   *Allium cepa*

Botanical information: A biennial plant of the *Lilaceae* family, and an extremely nutritious herb. It grows widely throughout Europe, Africa, America and Asia. The onion is a close relative of *Allium sativa* (Garlic) and both plants like a sheltered aspect with nutrient-rich soil.

Therapeutic uses: Primarily an antiseptic, but also a diuretic and expectorant. It contains a volatile oil, flavonoid glycosides, glucokinins and pectins.

The Czechoslovakian experts Doctors Frantisek Stary and Vaclav Jirasek in their book *Herbs – A Concise Guide In Colour,* describe the germicidal effects of the Onion as 'excellent', and it has long been used as an internal parasiticide and antiseptic.

An old folk-remedy for 'keeping germs at bay' suggests placing half an onion on the bedside table of a sickroom, and some years ago a large American university carried out tests to see whether there was any scientific basis to it. The researchers found that the Onion actually 'drew' airborne bacteria from the atmosphere and thus sanitized the sickroom.

When eaten, the Onion lowers blood-sugar levels significantly which has obvious therapeutic benefits.

Dosage: *Ad lib*.

Synonyms: Rounde Roote.

● **PARSLEY**   *Petroselinum crispum*

Botanical information: A biennial or perennial aromatic herb that was originally native to Europe but is now naturalized in most sub-tropical countries. It belongs to the *Umbelliferae* family.

Therapeutic uses: The therapeutic uses of Parsley can to some degree be explained by its rich nutrient content. The herb contains 8,230 I.U.s of vitamin A per 100gms; 193mgms of vitamin C, 4.3mgms of iron, 190mgms of calcium, 78mgms of potassium and 84mgms of phosphorus.

The rich mineral content is beneficial to the kidneys, particularly in cases of nephritis, and for several arthritic conditions.

The herb also has a powerful action on the urinary tract and female reproductive organs. The seeds of Parsley are strongly diuretic and are a common remedy for high blood-pressure. They are also, in the opinion of many experienced herbalists, a powerful emmenagogue that can be used to regulate the menses.

Dosage: ½–1 dr. of the liquid extract of the rootstock should be taken as prescribed.

Synonyms: Fairy Feathers.

● **PASSION FLOWER** *Passiflora incarnata*

Botanical information: The *Passiflorae* are a large genus of vines native to the South American countries. The flower gets its common name from the petals, stamens and sepals, which are supposed to represent the 'Christian cross' and various other aspects of Christ's impalement or 'passion'.

The fruit of the plant has a beautiful, exotic taste and is cultivated in New Zealand, Australia, South Africa and Hawaii.

Therapeutic uses: *P. incarnata* is not, contrary to popular belief because of its common name, an aphrodisiac; but it does have some medicinal virtues. Tablets containing the solid extract of the herb are popular in the U.K. as a mild sedative and nervine.

The plant can also be used as an anodyne, and may be employed in the treatment of neuralgia. One patient of mine suffered terribly from neuralgia and migraine and had tried several forms of alternative treatment including acupuncture and osteopathy, without success. As a last resort I prescribed Passiflora in tablet form. After four days the neuralgia pain went completely and she has not had a migraine attack since.

Dosage: 15 drops of the liquid extract, or the fruit may be eaten *ad lib*.

Synonyms: Maypops, Crown of Thorns.

● **PEACH** *Prunus persica*

Botanical information: The most widely cultivated fruit next to the apple, the peach was originally native to China but can now be found in North and South America, the Mediterranean area, Africa and Australia. The peach can also be grown in cooler climates under glass.

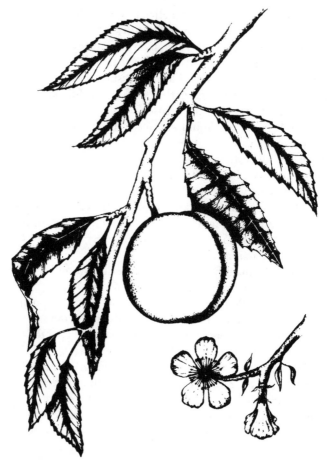

THE PEACH (*Prunus persica*) has been used since mediaeval times to treat whooping cough.

Therapeutic uses: As a nervine and tranquilizer: Oil of Peach (*Oleum persica*) has sedative properties and will relieve nervous tension and adverse stress reaction if taken on a regular basis over a prolonged period.

As an expectorant: The extract of the bark is mildly expectorant, but will work more efficiently if taken with *Sanguinaria canadensis* (Indian Red Paint or Bloodroot).

As a diuretic: A decoction of the bark makes a reasonably strong diuretic, but care should be taken as overuse can irritate the bladder.

John Gerard gave a marvellous description of the peach in his herbal, and captured its exquisite taste in the way that only the flowery diction of Mediaeval England could. 'The Peach tree' said Gerard 'is likewise a tree of no great bignesse . . . and these kindes of Peaches are very like to wine in taste, and therefore marvellous pleasant.'

Dosage: The fruit may be eaten *ad lib*, but the stones contain cyanogenetic glycosides and should NEVER be swallowed or left in the mouth for long periods.

Synonyms: Persica, Petch.

- **PELLITORY OFF THE WALL**   *Parietaria officinalis*

Botanical information: A quite widespread wild herb that grows most commonly in Europe and Great Britain. The plant flowers during June, July and early August.

Therapeutic uses: Popular in the South of France and in England as a remedy for all stones in the urinary tract, but particularly those found in the bladder. The plant is also mildly laxative.

Dosage: A tisane of Standard Strength.

Synonyms: Paritary, paritory, Pellitory Of The Wall.

- **PENNYROYAL**   *Mentha pulegium*

Botanical information: A lesser known species of mint, but one that grows commonly in the U.K. Culpeper noted that the herb could be found by 'the highways from London to Colchester' and Gerard that it 'groweth naturally wilde in moist and overflowne places, as in the Common neere London called Miles end.'

Therapeutic uses: For 'menstrual stoppage' as one Victorian pamphlet puts it, a tisane of Pennyroyal is said to be 'most efficacious', and several modern herbals recommend it for the treatment of amenorrhoea. Of course, the herb should never be taken during pregnancy in large doses because herbs that encourage the onset of menstruation invariably have abortifacient qualities in greater amounts.

Gerard suggested that it may be useful in cases of vertigo, or, if our modern medical parlance sounds a little dry, 'the swimming in the head and the paines and giddinesse thereof.'

Hill recommended it for whooping cough, directing that the expressed juice should be mixed with candy.

The oil of the Pennyroyal can be applied to the skin to ward off mosquitoes and other biting insects.

Dosage: Tisane of Standard Strength.

Synonyms: Pudding Grass, European Pennyroyal.

● **PEPPER** *Piper nigrum*

Botanical information: A woody, perennial vine that grows in the rain forests of South West India and is cultivated for its culinary value.

Therapeutic uses: A gastric tonic of the first order. Pepper is a powerful carminative that is particularly useful for removing gas from the gut, and taken with meals as a condiment it stimulates the production of gastric juices.

It has also been employed in cases of chills and influenza and seems to have a restorative action.

Dosage: Taken as desired as a condiment with food.

Synonyms: Black Pepper.

● **PEPPERMINT** *Mentha piperita*

Botanical information: Peppermint is a perennial hybrid of *M. aquatica* and *M. spicata*. It cannot really be described as a 'wild' plant in the true sense, but nevertheless, it can often be found in roadside ditches throughout the British Isles. The plant may be cropped twice, in June–July and during October.

Therapeutic uses: The plant is rich, up to 2%, in a volatile oil that contains bitters, tannins and the substance menthol.

Like most members of the Mint family, *M. piperita* is a tonic for the digestive system. It has both antiseptic and antispasmodic qualities which have caused it to be recommended by some herbalists for the treatment of peptic ulcers. Its aromatic property also makes it a useful aid to the digestion.

Peppermint has also been recognized by orthodox doctors as being useful in the treatment of some liver and gall-bladder disorders. It promotes the flow of bile and also helps to catabolize gall-stones.

American herbalists, taking a leaf from the book of the Pilgrim

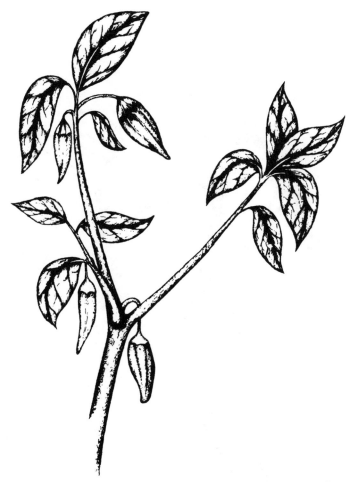

PEPPER (*Capsicum annuum*). A rich source of vitamin C, Pepper is used both as a gastric stimulant and as a remedy for allergies.

Fathers and the Amerindians who taught them, recommend that Peppermint is mixed with *Eupatorium perfoliatum* (Boneset) and *Salvia officinalis* (Sage) and taken as an expectorant and cough syrup.
Dosage: A tisane of Standard Strength and taken in 1 fl. oz. doses *pro re nata*.

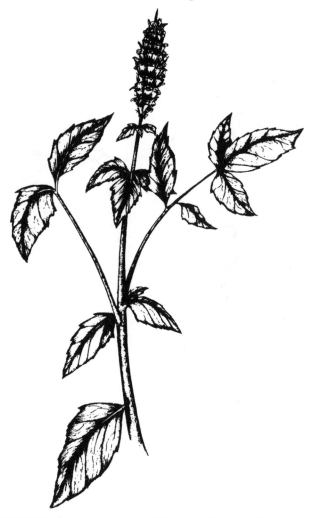

PEPPERMINT (*Mentha piperita*). Rich in the herbal oil menthol, Peppermint is used both as an aid to digestion and as an antiseptic for sore throats.

Synonyms: Pepper Mint, Brandy Mint, Balm Mint, American Mint, Lamb Mint, Curled Mint.

● **PILEWORT**   *Ranunculus ficaria*

Botanical information: A large genus of annuals and perennials more commonly called the Buttercups. There are over three hundred and twenty species, and although most are toxic to the human organism they do have therapeutic properties. *R. ficaria,* one of the better known of the Ranunculaceae medicinal herbs, is the one that concerns us specifically at this juncture.

Therapeutic uses: A herbal specific that is used to treat haemorrhoids (piles): distended varicose veins around the anus. The herb appears to be equally effective when taken internally as a tisane or applied externally in a balm or ointment.

Its efficacy is due to its astringency and extreme vasoconstrictive action, tightening up the blood vessels of the anus and thus shrinking the haemorrhoids.

Dosage: *PLEASE READ THIS SECTION CAREFULLY:* All species of Ranunculus contain the poisons protoanemonine and anemonal, including *R. ficaria.* Consquently the herb should NEVER be ingested fresh or rubbed on the skin where it may cause irritation. However, when the plant is dried the toxins break down into the reasonably innocuous substance anemonine. From this it can be seen that the plant should only be used AFTER drying. The tisane can be made to Standard Strength and taken 1–3 fl. oz. per day.

Synonyms: Lesser Celandine, Pile Buttercup.

● **PINKROOT**   *Spigelia marilandica*

Botanical information: A perennial of the *Loganiaceae* family which grows prolifically in certain areas of the U.S.A. The plant enjoys a nutrient rich soil and flourishes around Kentucky and other Eastern states, and in the South in Florida and Texas.

Therapeutic uses: Used exclusively as a vermifuge in the U.S.A. and in the majority of countries to which it is exported. The volatile alkaloids of *S. marilandica* have an extremely toxic effect upon intestinal parasites, and will quickly expel them from the intestine and bowel.

It is advisable to combine this herb with an efficient laxative, and this for two reasons. Firstly, it is possible that the volatile oils may irritate the intestines if they are allowed to stay in the digestive tract for an undue length of time. Secondly, the laxative action ensures that the worms are expelled from the bowel quickly and thus none are allowed to remain and recover, or possibly even breed. Both Wren and Kadans suggest Senna as the laxative of choice.

Dosage: 1 oz of the powdered root made into a tisane of Standard Strength. 1 tablespoon of the tisane should be taken in the morning and another on retiring. As little food as possible should be eaten during the day between the two dosages.

Synonyms: Wormgrass, American Wormroot, Carolina Pink, Spigelia, Maryland Pink, Maryland Pinkroot, Indian Pink, India Pink, Carolina Pinkroot.

● **PLANTAIN**   *Plantago major*

Botanical information: A perennial herb which flowers from May to September. It can be found throughout Europe including Scandinavia, Asia, Africa, the Americas, Australia and New Zealand.

Therapeutic uses: In ancient times the plant had a prominent place in many authorative herbals. Dioscorides and Pliny recommended it for, amongst other things, the treatment of malignant tumours, ulcers, bronchial disorders, fevers, infected wounds and bites, and also pustulous inflammatons.

In recent years the herb has been examined scientifically and found to be extremely useful in two main areas of treatment.

As an expectorant: Up to 10% of some parts of the plant may be mucilaginous, and this is aided by the glycoside aucubin to produce an expectorant action. So successful is the herb in remedying coughs and related bronchial/pulmonary ailments that several Russian pharmaceutical companies have invested large sums in having the plant cultivated so that they will have an adequate supply of its active ingredients.

As an external antiseptic: The plant has long been recognized as possessing antibiotic properties. Until the turn of the century Cumbrian farmers would apply the pulverized leaves of Plantain, along with a large pinch of salt, to rat–bites and other wounds that are potentially dangerous. Also, an old Romany remedy for boils suggests placing Plantain leaves over the pustulation.

Curiously, there is still confusion over exactly which of *P. Major's* chemical constituents imbues it with its antiseptic properties. As Flück says, some of its biochemicals are still 'little known'.

Dosage: Tisane of Standard Strength.

Synonyms: Ribwort, Ripple Grass.

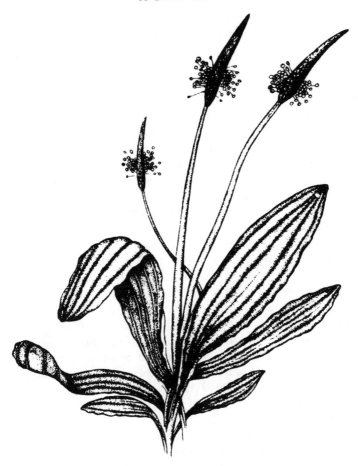

PLANTAIN (*Plantago major*) is popular in Eastern Europe as an expectorant.

● **PLEURISY ROOT** *Asclepias tuberosa*
Botanical information: A hardy, attractive, perennial shrub of the *Asclepiadaceae* family which grows in North, Central and South America.
Therapeutic uses: As you may have guessed, the root of *A. tuberosa* has been used successfully in the treatment of pleurisy. It regulates the breathing, reduces the temperature by acting as a diaphoretic and

also retards further inflammation of the pleura. The herb contains anodyne substances which also kill the pain to a certain extent.

The herb is widely available from herbal suppliers in the U.S.A., and is becoming an increasingly popular item amongst herbalists in the U.K. I recently purchased an ounce of high-quality root for just 36p.

Dosage: Tisane of Standard Strength taken three times a day.

Synonyms: Butterfly Weed, Swallow Wort, Swallowwort, Tuber Root, Wind Root, Pipple Root.

● **POKE ROOT** *Phytolacca decandra-americana*

Botanical information: There are around forty species of the *Phytolacca* genus, the majority being found in the U.S.A. The leaves of *most* (not all!) species are edible when cooked thoroughly, but they are extremely poisonous when raw.

P. decandra grows mainly in North America.

Therapeutic uses: Both the roots and berries can be used medicinally, although the roots have a stronger action. It is ranked alongside Sarsaparilla as an alterative in the U.S.A, as good a reference as any plant-medicine could hope to have, and it also seems to have anti-inflammatory properties. Indeed, it is particularly valued in the mountain state of Vermont as a cure for rheumatism.

Some herbalists recommend that the plant is useful in the treatment of various skin ailments, particularly those of an infectious nature such as scabies and *tinea* (ringworm). Its efficacy is probably exaggerated, but it has been used successfully in Canada in cases of psoriasis.

Dosage: The herb can be poisonous if taken or prescribed incorrectly. Only take as directed by a qualified practitioner.

Synonyms: Pocan, Pigeon Berry, Garget, Ink Berry.

● **PRICKLY ASH** *Zanthoxylum americana*

Botanical information: A temperate genus of trees and shrubs that inhabits Asia, Africa and the Americas. The North American species are those primarily used as medicines.

Therapeutic uses: *Z. americana* is often used in conjunction with another species: *Z. clavaherculis* (Southern Prickly Ash) as they have similar properties.

The bark contains stimulants that act as a general tonic and invigorator. It is a true alterative that can be employed in a variety of conditions, but notably in cases of glandular fever. (It also contains zanthoxylin which acts as a diaphoretic.)

The berries are similar to the bark in action, but as their active principles are more easily absorbed by the stomach they are considered stronger.

Dosage: ½–1 dr. of the fluid extract of the bark.

Synonyms: Toothache Tree, False Hercules, False Hercules Club, Yellowwood, Sootberry.

● **PRIMROSE** *Primulus vulgaris*

Botanical information: A well known species of the *Primulaceae* family which flowers from early March to mid April.

It is a common sight throughout the British Isles, and many of the five-hundred or so other species often form a pretty display along roadsides and in natural parkland areas.

Therapeutic uses: Like all members of the *Primulaceae* family, *P. vulgaris* is rich in glycosides. As we discussed in an earlier chapter, glycosides consist of several sugar parts and one non-sugar part. It is these non-sugar parts (or aglycones) in the *Primulaceae* that have a therapeutic action.

The plant has three uses: Firstly, it is extremely astringent and tends to reduce the severity of diarrhoea. It has also been used, again because of its astringency, in the treatment of internal bleeding, but with mixed results.

Secondly, the herb is rich in anodyne substances which give it both an antispasmodic and pain-killing quality. When taken as a tisane it eases pain in the stomach and intestines, and as a tincture it corrects cases of renal colic.

Thirdly, the herb can be employed as a vermifuge. Its action is not particularly strong, but it is valuable as part of a compound remedy.

Dosage: As directed by your practitioner.

Synonyms: Primula, Primuli.

● **PUMPKIN** *Cucurbita maxima*

Botanical information: Pumpkin is an edible fruit, though commonly called a vegetable in the culinary sense, of the *Cucurbita* genus. They are commonly eaten in the South of England, but more rarely in the North.

Therapeutic uses: The seeds of *C. maxima* are one of the most efficient vermifuges in the plant kingdom. They are particularly

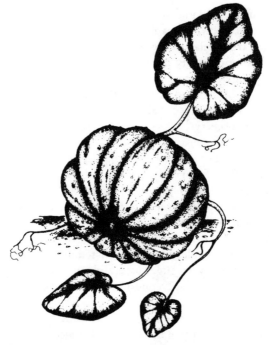

PUMPKIN (*Cucurbita maxima*) is used in the treatment of worms.

useful when the intestines are infected by the *taenia* or tapeworm.

For maximum effectiveness, the seeds must be taken in the correct manner. Various methods are suggested by different authorities, the following being the most sensible in my opinion:
Dosage: The patient must fast for twelve hours minimum, and then take a saline-based cathartic. This cleanses and disinfects the intestines of any remaining faecal matter, and also weakens the tapeworm.

2oz of the seeds are then crushed (not comminuted) and added to ¾ of a pint of milk that has been sweetened with ½ oz of honey and 1 oz of cane sugar.

⅓ of this mixture should be swallowed every 2–3 hours, and then, after the last dose, a moderate amount of Castor oil (oleum ricini) should be swallowed.
Synonyms: Whittington's Pouffé

● **QUASSIA** *Picraena excelsa*
Botanical information: A pan-American genus of trees and shrubs
that belongs to the *Simaroubaceae* family. *P. excelsa* and its related
species are used as ornamental trees in many parts of the tropics.
Therapeutic uses: Quassia chips: the yellowish chips of the Quassia
wood are still a common sight in herbal supply stores in many parts
of Latin America, and they have two main purposes: they are
anthelmintic and are frequently used as a home remedy for
pin-worms. Also, they contain potent bitter principles which act as a
stimulant to the digestion.
Dosage: A tincture can be prepared from the wood chips, but the
natives of Jamaica long ago devised another, rather ingenious
method. By carving cups and bowls from the wood, they furnished
themselves with drinking vessels that would impart the characteris-
tically bitter flavour of Quassia to any beverage that was poured into
them. Thus, water, beer and milk could be impregnated with
Quassia bitter principles and made more easily digestible. Quassia
should only be taken in small quantities.
Synonyms: Bitter Wood, Bitter Ash, Bitter Bark.

● **QUEEN'S DELIGHT** *Stillingia sylvatica*
Botanical information: The *Euphorbiaceae* family, to which the
Stillingia genus belongs, is an important botanical family which is
highly concentrated in the Americas, the Mediterranean countries
and Africa. *S. sylvatica:* a monoecious herb: grows profusely in the
United States, particularly around Virginia and the Florida coastline.
Therapeutic uses: In the U.K the herb is generally used as a laxative
which is also said to have blood-purifying properties. It has been
employed in syphilitic conditions with some success. Its use in this
regard tailed off here in the U.K. around the turn of the century, but
it was still prescribed regularly in the U.S.A until the 1950's.
    Both English and American herbalists have praised the herb for its
effectiveness in treating scrophula: a tuberculous infection of the
lymph glands of the neck.
    Its astringency has made it useful in the case of leucorrhoea, a
creamy-white discharge from the vagina (originating in the glands of
the cervix) which may be symptomatic of amenorrhoea or cervicitis.
Dosage: 2–5 grains of the solid ext.
Synonyms: Yaw Root, Silver Leaf, Queen's Root.

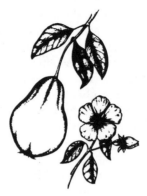

QUINCE (*Cydonia oblongata*) was used in ancient India as a treatment for Dysentry and certain eye diseases.

● **QUINCE** *Cydonia oblongata*
Botanical information: The *Cydonia* genus has only one species – C. *oblongata* – a deciduous tree native to Central Asia but now found in some areas of Europe and the U.S.A.

The fruit is edible, but its high acid content makes it extremely unpalatable. However, the fruit when ripe can be used to make jam or to flavour other cooked fruits.
Therapeutic uses: A weak, diluted expression (4 pts water to 1 pt liq. exp.) can be applied to dry, scaly skin and keens that appear on the digital extremities. A weaker solution (variable according to the condition) can be used as an eye lotion in cases of conjunctivitis and other eye ailments.
Dosage: The high acid content makes the taking of Quince unadvisable in the case of some gastric disorders. Check with your practitioner. As an external lotion, follow the formula above.
Synonyms: Cydonium, Quince Seed, Pyrus.
● **RED CLOVER** *Trifolium pratense*
Botanical information: An extremely common perennial herb found within the British Isles and Western Europe. It inhabits grasslands, roadsides, ditch and hedgebanks and will quickly follow the more pioneering herbs into freshly cultivated territory.

It lives comfortably in both dry soil and moist, and flowers

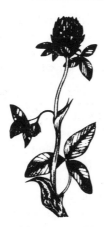

RED CLOVER (*Trifolium pratens*) is said by some to be effective in the treatment of cancer, although the orthodox medical profession as a whole has remained sceptical.

between May and Septembr. The herb is a close relative of *T. repens* (White or Dutch Clover).

Therapeutic uses: Over the years, a certain mystique has grown around *T. pratense* concerning its medicinal uses.

One of the most persistent rumours is that Red Clover is an effective anti-cancer treatment. Now let me say at this juncture that it is illegal for anyone other than a registered medical practitioner to claim that he or she can successfully treat cancer; however, it is acknowledged that some herbs do contain chemicals that can arrest the growth of certain kinds of tumour.

John Hoxey, a horse-breeder from Illinois, U.S.A., claimed in 1840 that several herbs – including Red Clover – had cured one of his prized Percheron horses of cancer. Scientific evidence over Hoxey's claim is conflicting. Orthodox critics have attempted to explain away the phenomenal number of successfully treated case-histories, but this can only be achieved by engaging in the most strenuous statistical acrobatics. An increasing number of herbalists are showing interest in the 'Hoxey herbs' and their claim for full clinical trials to be carried out would seem to be entirely justified.

Leaving the 'cancer cure' claims aside, Red Clover does have other uses. It is a bronchial sedative that effectively reduces coughing bouts, and some herbals even recommend it for whooping cough.

In Ireland an old remedy for winter colds was to drink Clover tea. It seems to have diaphoretic properties and acts as a restorative.

Dosage: A tisane of the petals of *T. pratense* may be taken freely.

WARNING: Some varieties of White or Dutch Clover contain the toxin *hydrocyanic acid*. *Cyanogenetic glycosides* can break down into prussic acid in the digestive system and prove extremely poisonous. Although only one death from Clover poisoning has ever been recorded (in New Zealand) incidents of toxicity occur regularly.

- **RHUBARB, ENGLISH**   *Rheum officinale*

Botanical information: *Rheum*, a genus of Asiatic perennials of the *Polygonaceae* family comprising of around fifty species. Some, like *R. rhabarbarum* (Garden Rhubarb) produce edible petioles. *R. officinale* is sometimes referred to as Medicinal Rhubarb.

Therapeutic uses: The laxative properties of *R. officinale* are notorious, although somewhat exaggerated. In moderate doses the herb acts as a non-purging aperient that is safe for children. Larger doses cause an evacuatory action.

It has other beneficial effects on the digestion too. It encourages the breakdown of carbohydrates by increasing salivation and stimulates bile production. It also acts as a vermifuge.

Rhubarb is quite nutritious. It contains vitamin A (30 I.U.s per 100 gms.), vitamin B complex, 9 mgs of vitamin C, 5 gms of protein, calcium, iron, phosphorous and potassium.

Dosage: As a foodstuff, but in moderation because of its laxative action. Rhubarb is also rich in oxalic acid and should therefore be avoided by those who suffer from arthritis (oxalic acid is a known aggravator). The leaves contain toxic soluble oxalates and should therefore not be eaten.

Synonyms: Rapontica, Raponticum.

- **ROSEMARY**   *Rosmarinus officinalis*

Botanical information: *Rosmarinus,* a small genus (4 species) of Mediterranean evergreens, is one of the most prized culinary herbs. It flowers from April to May, North of the Alps it is popular as an aromatic pot plant because of its beautiful aroma.

The Algerian varieties differ markedly from others and are described in some herbals as a different species.

Therapeutic uses: Like most of the aromatics, Rosemary increases the flow of digestive juices and acts as an aperient. It contains about 2% of essential oils and tannins which act as diuretics. Since Anglo-Saxon times the herb has been used to treat rheumatic conditions, and herbalists today prescribe it for neuritis, neuralgia and similar ailments.

Oil of Rosemary can be massaged into the joints of arthritic patients to produce similar pain-killing effects. It has also been prescribed in cases of migraine.

Rosemary is a popular ingredient in shampoos and hair tonics. It emoliates and sooths the scalp, reducing the tendency of the dermis to flake and produce dandruff. Some herbalists hold that premature balding can be arrested by applying Oil of Rosemary to the scalp, but to my knowledge there is no clinical evidence to support this theory.

Dosage: A weak tisane of Rosemary (½ oz. of the comminuted herb to 1 pint of water) can be taken in moderation. The oil can be applied externally as required.

Synonyms: Rose Mary.

● **RUE** *Ruta graveolens*

Botanical information: Rue is a European perennial that flowers from June to early September. The *Ruta* genus is of the *Rutaceae* family.

It grows mainly in Southern Europe and prefers an elevated climate. It does not require particularly nutritious soil (providing it is alkaline) but prefers rocky, limestone slopes that are not waterlogged.

Therapeutic uses: The chemical make-up of the plant is interesting. It contains traces (0.1 – 0.2%) of an essential oil, furocoumarins, bitters, resins, tannins and other biochemical ingredients.

The crude drug is a vasodilator and increases the flow of blood to the muscular tissue. It is also a powerful emmenagogue that can be used in cases of amenorrhoea.

A weak tisane can be used as an opthalmicum. According to Gerard and others, it will 'quicken the sight' and 'greatly improve the vision'.

Rue also has styptic properties. In times past the powdered herb was inhaled through the nostrils to stop nose-bleeds, but it must be said that no competent herbalist today would recommend this treatment unless the patient was strictly supervised. Rue has hallucinogenic properties when inhaled in large amounts and dosages must be strictly controlled.

Dosage: 20 grains can be taken under supervision, but the herb should not be used at all during pregnancy as it is an abortifacient. Large doses taken orally produce the aforementioned hallucinations and also violent retching.

Synonyms: Garden Rue, Yellow Rue, Roe, Herb Grace, Ave-Grace.

● **RUPTUREWORT** *Herniaria glabra*

Botanical information: An annual or perennial herb that flowers from late May to mid September. It can be found throughout all the temperate regions of Europe, the Mediterranean and Western Asia, but favours a lowland elevation with dry, stony ground with an alkaline soil. The plant is well localized in Europe but has never been cultivated successfully.

Therapeutic uses: A G.P. whom I know once told me that the idea of a herb being useful in the treatment of just one ailment was preposterous. He seemed to think that we herbalists have a vision of the Creator fashioning *H. glabra* and then saying 'There now, and while we're at it let's make it useful for treating hernias'. Of course, I, even as a committed Christian, find that idea preposterous also, but it is a curious fact that the chemical make-up of Rupturewort does make it useful for treating ruptures. To establish why, it is useful to know a few snippets of information about the herb's history as a medicine.

Almost all the major herbals recommend it for the treatment of prostate inflammation, ruptures, bladder infection etc. Gerard, to quote but one, said that it was 'good for Ruptures' and that 'very many that have beene bursten were restored to health by the use of this herbe'. Gerard also recommends Crane's Bill (another herb for the treatment of ruptures) and some authorities recommend that the two are best taken together.

There is certainly no mystique about its efficacy:

1) It has a diuretic effect and thus reduces the number of bacteria in the bladder. It also prevents pain in the bladder and ureters because it

is an antispasmodic. Interestingly, the diuretic effect encourages the expulsion of sodium and urea but does not increase the volume of urine.

2) The herb contains coumarins and flavones which seem to play some part in reducing the inflammation of the prostate gland, toning up muscle tissue and encouraging the flow of oxygenated blood to the herniated area.

3) The glycoside herniarine acts as an anodyne and relieves the pain of an infected urinary system or prostate gland.

Dosage: A tisane made to Standard Stength and taken in wineglass-full doses three times a day. Best taken under the guidance of a practitioner.

Synonyms: Herniary, Breastwort, Breast Wort.

● **SAFFLOWER** *Carthamus tinctorius*

Botanical information: A genus of herbaceous plants cultivated in the U.S.A., Mexico, India and Eurasia (also to a lesser extent in Southern and Central Europe).

There are about fifteen species of *Cathamus,* a genus of the *Compositae* family.

Therapeutic uses: The seeds and kernel of the Safflower are rich in a fixed oil (25% and 50% respectively) and are widely heralded as a preventative medicine, particularly in the prevention of heart disease. Safflower effectively lowers the level of cholesterol in the bloodstream.

The oil has a soothing effect upon the intestines. It is also a laxative, but does not work by irritant action.

Dosage: The flowerheads can be made into a weak tisane (⅓ oz to 1 pint of water), but neither large amounts of the tisane nor the seeds should be taken during pregnancy as they are potentially abortifacient.

Synonyms: American Saffron, Trist Saffron, False Saffron, Bastard Saffron, Dyers' Saffron, Flores Catharmi.

● **SARSAPARILLA** *Smilax aristolochioefolia*

Botanical information: The *smilax* genus contains several species of Sarsaparilla, and some confusion exists between them and other unrelated species which also bear the common name Sarsaparilla.

S. aristolochioefolia is a true Sarsaparilla and the one that most herbalists in the U.K. recognize. In the United States however, the herb *Aralia nudicaulis* (American Sarsaparilla) is extrmely popular and is often referred to simply as 'Sarsaparilla'. Thus British herbalists, when reading American herbal literature, often confuse the two. Some English herbals have even referred to *S. aristolochioefolia* as *American* Sarsaparilla because the herb grows profusely in the Latin American countries, but whilst this common name may be geographically correct it is nevertheless misleading. *A nudicaulis* is the only species that can correctly be called American Sarsaparilla.

Schisandra coccinea, Hardenbergia violacea and *Hemidesmus indicus* are also called by the common name Sarsaparilla in some areas.

Therapeutic uses: The herb is an excellent blood-purifier and alterative. It is frequently used in the treatment of all infectious diseases where the blood shows some abnormal quality.

The Aztecs used this herb in the treatment of syphilis, chronic skin ailments (particularly those that cause putrid ulceration of the dermis) and in cases of bone disease.

The plant is used in Britain as a tonic and restorative, Again, its antiseptic qualities have been recognized, as they were by the Amerindians, and a decoction of the herb is often used as a treatment for ringworm and parasitic skin infections.

Its restorative powers are particularly useful in the treatment of influenza. *S. aristolochioefolia* is a powerful diaphoretic and if it is taken just before going to bed it will cause profuse perspiration.

Dosage: A decoction of 1 oz. of the powdered root in 1 pint of water. 1 tablespoonful of the liquid to be taken frequently.

Synonyms: Bamboo Brier, Vera Cruz, Small Spikenard, Wild Sasp, Chinese Root, China Root.

- **SASSAFRAS** *Sassafras albidum*

Botanical information: A small genus of deciduous trees that consists of three species (one in North American and Canada and two in Eastern Asia) that are distinctive because of their aromatic wood, bark and root.

S. albidum, the American species, is a valuable source of income to those who cultivate it. It is used by parfumery houses as an aromatic additive, by food manufacturers as a flavouring agent and by pharmaceutical companies as a source of antiseptic oils.

The word Sassafras comes from the Roman *saxum* (stone) and *frangere* (break). This is because the powerful roots of *S. albidum* can grow in between rock strata and break them open.

Therapeutic uses: As a diaphoretic: Sassafras wood, normally sold in chips like Cassia, can be made into a tisane and taken to induce diaphoresis. It is reported that rheumatic patients gain considerable relief by taking the herb as a tisane. The greater the diaphoretic effect the more the pain seems to be relieved.

As a stimulant: The herb is a mild stimulant that has a similar action to caffeine.

As a diuretic: A tisane of the herb is mildly diuretic. A stronger diuretic draught can be made by decoction.

As a remedy for skin ailments: The tisane can be used as a skin lotion for psoriasis and related conditions.

Dosage: A tisane of Standard Strength; or the oil can be taken three drops at a time as directed by your practitioner. The leaves are used by the Amerindians to make soup.

Synonms: Ague Tree, Saxifrax, Mitten Tree, Cinnamon Wood, Gumbo.

- **SCULLCAP**   *Scutellaria laterifolia*

Botanical information: A genus of three hundred species of the *Labiatae* family that can be found in virtually every country of the world except South Africa.

S. laterifolia grows in the U.S.A. where its medicinal virtues were first discovered.

Therapeutic uses: Almost universally acknowledged to be the finest nervine in the therapeutic armoury of the herbal practitioner. It is an excellent remedy for all types of nervous complaint, and also for both reactive and endogenous depression.

Small doses of *S. laterifolia* have been of benefit in cases where the following symptoms were present:

> nervous spasms
> tension headaches
> muscular tremors
> arrythmia
> sleeplessness
> irritability
> St. Vitus' dance (chorea)
> Parkinsonism

One other symptom that has been treated successfully with Scullcap is hydrophobia: a morbid fear of water. Hydrophobia is also one of the classic symptoms of the dreaded disease rabies, and some herbals have suggested that *S. laterifolia* can be used as a treatment not just for the hydrophobia but also for rabies itself. Let me set matters straight. *There is no clinical evidence that Scullcap can reverse the progress of the disease or in any way improve the prognosis for a rabid patient.*

Some Canadian varieties of *S. laterifolia* are particularly astringent, and Canadian herbalists occasionally apply the liquid extract of the herb to open wounds to promote a rapid healing of the tissues.

Dosage: A tisane of Standard Strength taken frequently (½ cup every three hours).

Synonyms: Quaker's Hat, Quaker's Bonnet, Madderweed, Mad Weed, Skullcap.

• **SCURVY GRASS**   *Cochlearia officinalis*

Botanical information: A genus of Cruciferous annuals and perennials that thrive in the arctic and alpine Northern Hemisphere. They grow in abundance near coastal areas and at the foot of inland mountain ranges and plateaux.

In the U.K., Culpepper noted that the herb could be found near the river Thames, along the Essex and Kentish shores and near several of the seaports.

Scurvy Grass is sometimes called Spoonwort because of the concave nature of its leaves, and some authorities (Spooner and Lust) suggest that it may be the *herb britannica* mentioned by the ancient Greeks.

Therapeutic uses: No prize for guessing, of course, that the herb has been used successfully in the treatment of scurvy – a skin condition caused by a nutritional deficiency of vitamin C. Scurvy Grass contains two biochemicals which make it useful in treating this ailment. Firstly, it contains some vitamin C (although not a tremendous amount), and secondly, it is rich in potash salts which are extremely beneficial in the case of some skin diseases.

Captain Cook was the first person to use *C. officinalis* in the treatment of scurvy on a wide basis. During his voyages in the Southern Seas he became concerned at the disastrous effect that scurvy was having upon the crew. He ordered them to take a beverage made from the herb which was quite successful.

Culpepper said; 'infused, or the juice expressed, it is better than a decoction, because the volatile parts are lost in boiling; it is a specific remedy against scurvy; it purfies the body from the bad effects of the distemper and clears the skin of scabs, pimples and foul eruptions.'

Dosage: A strong tisane (2 oz of the herb to 1 pint of water) should be taken in wineglass-full doses six times a day.

Synonyms: Spoonwort, Carnson, Skeewort, Erba a Cucchiaino, Coclearia, Skeawyrt.

- **SELF-HEAL** *Prunella vulgaris*

Botanical information: *P. vulgaris* is one of several species of *Prunella* which grow throughout Europe, Africa, Asia and the Americas. It is usually found in woods and forests and near natural windbreaks that afford it some protection.

The herb flowers from late March until May, and is picked when the flowers are at their best in April. However, the flowers are not the parts used (the herb contains the therapeutic properties): it is simply that the active principles are found in greater amounts when the herb is flowering.

Therapeutic uses: An extremely astringent agent. Self-Heal contains tannins and other astringent agents which have proved useful in the case of certain infections. The liquid expression of the herb draws tissues together and creates an unfavourable environment for alien bacteria. It has been used most successfully in mouth and throat infections.

William Coles, in his comprehensive herbal, said that *P. vulgaris* was a marvellous remedy for 'an extraordinary inflammation or swelling, as well as in the mouth or throat'.

Its action on the digestive system is also beneficial. It soothes the inflamed mucous membranes after digestive disturbances have occurred, and stops diarrhoea efficiently.

The refined drug was once injected intravenously to relieve hypertension and intracranial pressure, but this practice is no longer carried out.

Dosage: A tisane of Standard Strength, taken 1 fl oz every four hours.

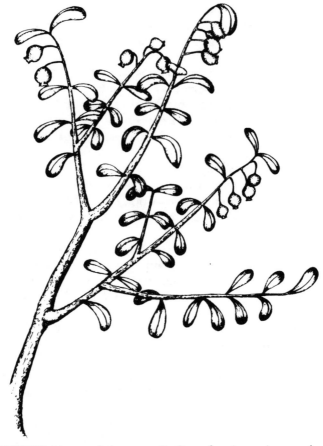

BEARBERRY (*Arctostaphylos uva-ursi*). One of an increasing number of herbs that are being cultivated in the Soviet Union for their medicinal properties. Bearberry has a strong disinfectant action.

Synonyms: Heal-All, Heal-Self, Hook-Heal, Siclewort, Sicle-Wort, Sicklewort.

● **SHEPHERD'S PURSE**   *Capsella bursa-pastoris*
Botanical information: There are several species of *Capsella*, the best known of which is *C. bursa-pastoris*. It grows almost worldwide, unlike its relative species which are confined to Southern Europe and several parts of Russia.

Shepherd's Purse will adapt to most soil types, but prefers a rich, loamy, well watered location. It flowers and fruits throughout the year, and just one plant can produce fifty thousand seeds in a season.

Fernie said 'This herb is of natural growth in most parts of the world, but varies in luxuriance according to soil and situation. Whilst thickly strewn over the whole surface of the earth, it faces alike the heat of the tropics and the rigours of the Arctic regions; even if trodden underfoot it rises again and again with ever-enduring vitality, as if designed to fulfil some special purpose in the far-seeing economy of nature.'

Therapeutic uses: Shepherd's Purse contains the amine called choline which acts as a vasoconstrictor.

A tisane of the herb will cause blood vessels and muscular tissue to contract, and has been used to hasten parturition during childbirth by causing womb contractions.

It has a powerful styptic action that has proved useful in cases of menorrhagia and other abnormal uterine haemorrhages. (Of course, all abnormal bleeding from the vagina should receive prompt medical attention.)

During World War 1, most haemostats were produced from *Hydrastis canadensis* (Golden Seal). Due to the war situation, the plant became in rather short supply between 1914–1917, and so alternative haemostats and styptics were produced from *C. bursa-pastoris*.

Dosage: A tisane should be taken at Standard Strength, one wineglass-full three times a day.

Synonyms: Shepherd's Sprout, Permacety, Mother's Heart, Pick-Purse, Pick-Pocket, Toy-Wort, Clapper's Pouch, Casewort, Rattle Pouch.

● **SLIPPERY ELM** *Ulmus fulva*

Botanical information: One of the thirty-four species of Elm tree. It grows in the U.S.A.; particularly in the Central and Northern states. It is often found near Dakota and most parts of Florida.

Therapeutic uses: Some herbals record that *U. fulva* is the only species of Elm to have medicinal qualities. This is not quite true, but it is correct to say that, of all the Elms, *U. fulva* is by far the most therapeutically useful.

The Amerindians have made great use of *U. fulva,* probably more than any other race. Since time immmemorial they have used the ground, inner bark of the tree to make a beverage that is both soothing to an inflamed alimentary canal and also very nutritious. The herb contains an abundance of tannins and mucilagens which are both astringent and anti-inflammatory. When the comminuted bark is taken with milk it lines the gut and intestines and protects the mucous membranes from irritation.

I spoke to one of the directors of Arun Products Ltd of Croyden who market the famous *Thompson's Slippery Elm Food.* How did Mr. Ford rate Slippery Elm? 'I was brought up with it', he told me. 'I well remember the days when it was commonly used as a baby-food and as a remedy for digestive disorders.'

It must be said at this point that neither Mr. Ford or any other director of Arun foods makes any claims regarding the medicinal value of their product. 'We market our product as a food', said Mr. Ford, 'NOT a medicine.' The packaging of *Thompson's Slippery Elm Food* avoids any claims of therapeutic value, but few herbalists would deny that *Ulmus fulva* is one of the finest remedies for digestive disorders in the plant kingdom.

Dosage: One or two heaped teaspoonfuls of the comminuted bark should be added to a little milk and made into a paste. This should then be topped up with hot milk and stirred before drinking. Add honey to taste.

Synonyms: Moose Elm, Elm, Oohooskah, Red Elm, Ulmenrinde, Ecorce d'Orme.

● **SNAKE ROOT** *Aristolochia reticulata* Botanical information: There are approximately three-hundred and fifty species of *Aristolochia* and several carry the common name Snake Root. They grow in abundance in the U.S.A. where they are prized for their medicinal qualities. *A. reticulata* and the other Aristolochia species belong to the *Aristolochiaceae* family.

Therapeutic uses: *A. reticulata* has quite a few therapeutic uses. It is recommended as a diaphoretic, tonic, nervine, anodyne and antibiotic.

It is held to be valuable in the treatment of typhoid and malaria, and can be taken internally when other remedies such as *Myroxylon pereirae* (Peruvian Bark) may cause digestive problems as a side-effect of taking large doses.

Some American herbals recommend *A. reticulata* for the treatment of bilious conditions, but it is likely that they are confusing this herb with a related species: *A. serpentaria* (Virginia Snakeroot), which is of great value in treating liver and gall-bladder disorders.

Dosage: A weak tisane made from ½ oz of the powdered herb to 1 pint of water. One tablespoonful to be taken three to five times a day.

Synonyms: Red River Snakeroot, Texas Snakeroot, Serpentary, Texan Root.

● **SORREL** *Rumex acetosa*

Botanical information: The *Rumex* genus contains a large variety of medicinal plants, usually referred to as docks or sorrels.

R. acetosa is a perennial herb that flowers during June and can be found throughout the British Isles and Europe. It thrives in salt-marshes and moist meadowland and often grows by roadsides.

Therapeutic uses: Used internally as a febrifuge and externally as a refrigerant.

Internally, the herb has a cooling action that is said to nullify the effects of sunstroke and exhaustion. Externally, the leaves may be laid on bruises and inflammations in poultice form.

In France the herb is eaten as a vegetable (boiled like spinach) and used to make Sorrel sauce, a garnish for meat dishes. Gerard said that Sorrel sauce 'is the best, not onely in vertue, but also in the pleasantnesse of his taste.'

The French herbalists also value Sorrel as a remedy for anaemia as it is rich in iron.

Dosage: Large amounts of Sorrel can be dangerous as the leaves contain quite high levels of soluble oxalates. Unfortunately the symptoms of toxicity may not become fully evident until twelve hours or more after the herb is ingested. Sheep are the most common victims, but poisoning in humans is not unknown.

Synonyms: Alazan, Alazar, Acetosa.

● **SPEARMINT** *Mentha spicata*

Botanical information: *M. spicata* is the most commonly cultivated of the various *Mentha* species. It is indigenous to Europe and North Africa, but now grows widely in Asia, America, and also in the British Isles where it was introduced by the Romans.

The herb likes damp, peaty soil that is nutrient-rich and not too exposed to the elements.

Therapeutic uses: Despite the fact that Spearmint is closely related to

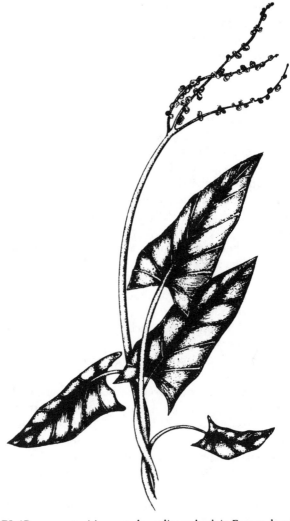

SORREL (*Rumex acetosa*) is a popular culinary herb in France, but it can also be used in a medical context to treat fevers.

Peppermint its chemical constituents are somewhat different. For one thing, the plant contains no menthol, but instead is rich in another volatile oil called carvone (also present in *Carum carvi* or

Caraway).

Like *M. piperita*, *M. spicata* is used by herbalists as a carminative. I can't quote any scientific papers to back up my claim, but my clinical experience tells me that Spearmint is far more effective than other members of the mint family in treating digestive disorders. Its carminative and stimulant action is more efficient, and, unlike some related species, *M. spicata* does not produce feelings of nausea when taken in large amounts.

Both Parkinson and Ceres recommend that the herb be applied externally for the relief of skin ailments. Parkinson says that a decoction of mint can be used as a lotion for children whose hands are covered in scabs and blotches. Ceres commends it for inflammation of the vaginal membrane and pruritus.

Dosage: Tisane of Standard Strength.

Synonyms: Lady's Garden, Mackerel Herb.

- **SQUILL** *Scilla maritima*

Botanical information: The species of the Scilla (Squill) genus grow commonly in the Mediterranean countries and are members of the Lilaceae family. There are three main species; *S. autumnalis* (Autumn Squill), *S. natalensis* (Blue Squill) and the medicinal species *S. maritima*.

Red or Algerian squill is used as an ingredient in rodent pesticides.

Therapeutic uses: Squill has a long history as a medicine. It was known to Hippocrates, Pliny, Dioscorides and Avicenna as well as other medical notables.

The herb is rich in cardiac glycosides which were (and occasionally still are) used to stimulate heart activity. It also acts as a diuretic which may help to reduce blood-pressure, thus indirectly helping cardiac action in another way.

The herb is also an expectorant which is of benefit in certain bronchial and pulmonry disorders.

Dosage: The plant is a violent poison that causes a drastic evacuation of the bowel and uncontrollable retching. It should only be prescribed by qualified herbalists in minute, carefully monitored dosages.

Synonyms: Poison Bush.

- **STAR ANISE** *Illicum verum*

Botanical information: *Illicium* is an Asiatic genus of evergreens commonly referred to as Aniseed Trees. They are to be found in the Americas (particularly North America) and also in the West Indies and their native Asia.

Star Anise is indigenous to China and is perhaps the most valuable species. The extract is used to flavour soft drinks and candy and the seeds yield a medicinal oil of great potency.

Therapeutic uses: A carminative with a similar action to *Pimpinella anisum* (Anise Seed), Star Anise is often added to commercial preparations sold for the relief of flatulence and 'wind pains' in young babies.

The herb also has antibacterial properties which have been used successfully in the treatment of *streptococcal* infections.

Dosage: As a tisane of Standard Strength. Only toxic in large doses.

Synonyms: Chinese Anise, Chinese Aniseed.

● **TAMERIND**   *Tamarindus indica*

Botanical information: A tree of the *Leguminosae* family that grows in India and is cultivated for its edible fruits. The fruit itself is not eaten whole, but the acidic pap is used as an ingredient in Asian dishes.

Therapeutic uses: Tamerind is a quite nutritious foodstuff. Although its vitamin content is not spectacular (30 I.U.s of vitamin A per 100 gms, a generous helping of the B complex, 2 mgs of vitamin C), it also contains 3 mgs of protein, 62 gms of carbohydrate, 73mgs of iron and 113 mgs of phosphorus. It has a calorific value of 240.

A drink can be made (see notes on dosage) from the pap and used as a febrifuge and restorative. It also acts as a laxative and can be used – depending on the dosage given – as a mild aperient or a purgative.

Dosage: A tisane can be made by using 1oz of the pap to 1 qt of water.

If the same amount of pap is boiled with 2 pints of milk the result is a slightly viscous liquid called Tamerind whey or Tamerind milk.

Synonyms: Tamarind.

● **TOBACCO**   *Nicotiana rustica*

Botanical information: The *nicotiana* genus contains the most notorious (and yet the most popular) plant poison in the world: Tobacco. Two species: *N. tabacum* and *N. rustica*: are cultivated on a colossal basis for the Tobacco-smoking market. The plant is extremely addictive and causes physical (also psychological) dependency within a short space of time.

Therapeutic uses: When one considers the disastrous harm that tobacco causes to the lungs and heart of people who smoke the stuff it is difficult to believe that it can be of any therapeutic benefit. And yet it most certainly is, as many 19th century American cowhands would testify were they alive today. More will be said about the toxic effects of Tobacco under 'dosage', but the alkaloids have an antiseptic nature which caused many American cowboys to use the leaves in a 'Tobacco poultice' which was applied to any horse or beast that might have developed a tumour or ulcer on its leg. Quite often, the swelling would simply disappear.

Italian Gypsies also used Tobacco to heal wounds. They would spit on the cut or abrasion and then lie some dried Tobacco leaves across the top, binding them in place with a clean rag.

The value of Tobacco as a healing agent cannot really be disputed, but as there are many other herbs which are just as beneficial but without being so toxic, I cannot see that it's use would be regularly warranted.

Dosage: Tobacco taken raw (or in a tisane) is a most efficient poison. The alkaloids cause vomiting, convulsions and respiratory failure in even minute doses.

If Tobacco were to be placed across a large, open wound, it is possible that enough toxin could be absorbed into the bloodstream to cause poisoning.

Synonyms: Tobacca.

● **UVA URSI**   *Arctostaphylos uva-ursi*

Botanical information: A genus of American shrubs that belongs to the *Ericaceae* family. There are over seventy species, Uva Ursi being the one with the most pronounced medicinal qualities.

The fruit of *A. uva-ursi* formed part of the staple diet of the early American settlers, being introduced to them by the local indian tribes.

Therapeutic uses: A popular astringent and diuretic amongst herbalists in the U.S.A., Uva Ursi is used almost exclusively in the treatment of urinary disorders. If we can believe the reports of sundry practitioners around the globe, the herb will act as an anthilic, quickly breaking down kidney and bladder stones and, if taken as a preventative medicine, stop new ones forming. It has also been recommended for ulceration of the bladder and leucorrhoea, and to reduce an excessive discharge of menstrual blood.

Dosage: Tisane of Standard Strength taken four times a day, one wineglass-full at a time.

Synonyms: Barberry (not to be confused with *Berberis vulgaris,* also called Barberry), Mountain Box, Rockberry, Upland Cranberry.

● **VALERIAN**   *Valeriana officinalis*

Botanical information: A genus of perennial herbs that can be found distributed throughout most of the temperate regions. *V. officinalis* flowers from May to September and grows abundantly in moist meadowland and on herbaceous slopes.

The herb is cultivated in Germany, Holland, Belgium and the U.S.S.R. for pharmaceutical purposes.

Therapeutic uses: Valerian contains a variety of potent principles including the valepotriates, some spasmolytics, an essential oil, bitter principles and the depressant bornyl valerate.

The herb was first mentioned in a medicinal context by Isaac Judaeus in the year 924 A.D., and has since been held in high regard by master herbalists as a fine nervine and sedative.

Dioscorides taught that it was an antidote for poisons; Gerard quoted Dioscorides and recommended it for the same. But it is as a treatment for nervous complaints that Valerian has become noteworthy. Nervous spasms and tremors, phobias, insomnia and restlessness may be helped by the careful prescription of Valerian.

A colleague of mine has had some success in treating the condition known as Ekbom's Syndrome (or 'restless legs') with a tincture of Valerian root. This condition, which probably sounds rather absurd unless you happen to suffer from it, causes the person to feel that they must constantly move their legs to prevent cramp. The symptoms usually intensify at night when the person is in a supine position. A tisane of Valerian root will normally keep the symptoms at bay if taken on a regular basis after the initial course of treatment is over.

Dosage: Valerian is not addictive or habit-forming and causes no known side-effects. However, it should not be taken in large doses except under supervision. A tisane of Standard Strength should be made.

Synonyms: Setwall, Set-Wall, Great Valerian, Valeriana.

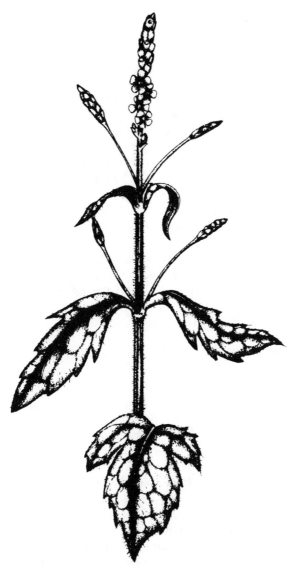

VERVAIN (*Verbena hastata*) is a popular folk-remedy for colds, but is also used in the treatment of nervous disorders, and even epilepsy.

- **VERVAIN**   *Verbena officinalis*

Botanical information: A varied genus of American shrubs that are used extensively by parfumery houses because of their delicate aroma. The species *V. officinalis* (*Verbenaceae* family) is now naturalized to Britain. Culpeper states that the herb can be found under hedges, by waysides and on 'other waste grounds'; Gerard that it grows in 'untilled places neere unto hedges, high-waes and commonly by ditches almost every where'.

The word Vervain is of Celtic origin and means 'driving away' or 'scaring off'. The name is said to indicate its medicinal use of 'driving away' certain diseases. Others interpret the words more precisely, pointing out that not only does the first syllable 'fer' mean 'driving away' but that the second syllable 'faen' means 'stone'. This strongly suggests that the ancient Celts were aware of the herb's anthilic properties.

Therapeutic uses: Gerard gives an interesting treatise on Vervain in his herbal, and whilst he recommends it for the 'Tertian and Quartaine Fevers', he derides those who in his day promoted the herb as a cure for the plague. 'These men are deceived' he charged 'because instead of a good and sure remedy they minister no remedy at all.'

The herb is generally employed as a diaphoretic or sudorific in cases of chills and colds. It has a quite pleasant, invigorating action and also helps clear blocked nasal passages.

The herb is also known to have antidepressant qualities. This idea goes back to Pliny at least and does have some scientific validity. However, its Sedative action is weak unless taken in quite large doses.

The American *V. hastata* (Blue Vervain) is regarded by many as a variety of *V. officinalis*. It is used to treat pleurisy and has an expectorant principle that can be of value in other pulmonary isorders.

Dosage: Taken in large doses the herb is poisonous. ½ dr. of the fluid extract should be taken as prescribed by your practitioner, or a tisane of Standard Strength can be taken 1 fl oz five times a day.

Synonyms: Wild Hyssop, Verbina, Devil's Medicine, Bastard Balm.

- **WITCH HAZEL**   *Hamamelis virginiana*

Botanical information: There are five species of Witch Hazel, all deciduous trees native to Eurasia and the Americas. The main pharmaceutical source of the plant is in the U.S.A. where it inhabits the damp woodlands and swamps around Florida and Minnesota.

Therapeutic uses: *H. virginiana* is now only rarely taken internally as a herbal medicine, but it is becoming increasingly popular as an external refrigerant and antiseptic lotion. The leaves and bark contain essential oils and tannins which are effective in reducing the inflammation of boils, cuts, and other localized skin eruptions.

In hospitals the distilled extract of Witch Hazel is often applied in a cold compress to delicate tissue (such as the scrotum sac) that has become inflamed for some reason, and to haemorrhoids because of its astringent action.

Witch Hazel can also be used as an enema for internal haemorrhoids or, more commonly, the active principle *hamamelin* is added to suppositories.

Dosage: The distilled extract may be applied as a refrigerant lotion.

Synonyms: Spotted Elder, Spotted Alder, Winter Bloom, Striped Elder, Bending Elder, Snapping Hazel, Snapping Hazelnut, Tobacco Wood.

● **YELLOW DOCK**   *Rumex crispus*

Botanical information: A large genus of the *Polygonaceae* family that grows in nearly all the temperate regions, but R. crispus is mainly restricted to the British Isles and Western Europe.

The herb grows on wasteland, near hedges, as a weed in urban areas and in small woods, but dislikes montane elevations, exposed moors and heaths. Its small red-to-brown flowers appear in June and last till October/November.

Therapeutic uses: The leaves of the Yellow Dock are sometimes used as an antidote to nettle stings, the leaf being rubbed over the affected area. It must be said however that the Broad Leaved Dock (Rumex obtusifolium) has a more efficient action in this respect.

Internally the root may be taken as a laxative and is also said to be beneficial for some skin diseases like cystic acne.

Dosage: The leaves of Dock contain soluble oxalates and are extremely poisonous. They should only be used externally.

A tisane can be made from the comminuted root at Standard Strength and taken as prescribed by your practitioner.

Synonyms: Curled Dock, Sad Dock.

3   Poisonous Plants

Serious toxicity from swallowing poisonous plant material is a relatively rare event, but of course, 'relatively rare' is still not good enough. Every year, several amateur herbalists poison themselves (or even worse someone else) by ingesting poisonous plants or 'prescribing' them for a friend.

Many colleges and faculties that teach herbal medicine as a profession include in their text material a 'Poisons List' which is, quite simply, a shortlist of herbs that should never be taken internally under any circumstances. These lists vary from one faculty to another, and of course from one country to another, and I have never seen one that is totally inclusive. Given our lack of knowledge concerning many herbs it is unlikely that a comprehensive list could be produced at this juncture.

Many of the plants mentioned in this 'Concise Herbal' are admittedly poisonous, and where documented evidence regarding their toxicity has been available I have included a warning in the text, normally under the DOSAGE heading. But the reader must remember that many herbs *have not had their biochemical qualities, both toxic and therapeutic, fully documented.* Thus it must be said that no herb should EVER be taken in even small amounts unless you are totally familiar with it. Before you take a medicinal herb, read every word that you can about it in your collection of herbal and botanical literature. Alternatively, seek out the advice of a seasoned practitioner.

If Poisoning Does Occur

If the victim has swallowed an unidentified *fungus* (toadstool, mushroom etc.), ALWAYS induce vomiting as quickly as possible and then telephone the doctor.

If the victim has *just* swallowed some toxic plant material, induce

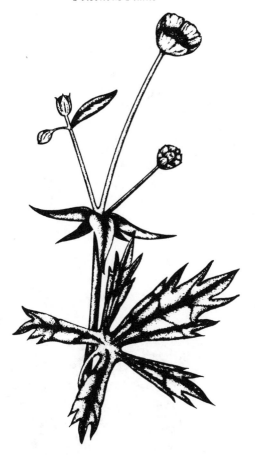

COMMON BUTTERCUP (*Ranunculus acris*) may be used medicinally, but only by experts and after drying as it contains an extremely poisonous sap.

vomiting if possible. However, if the victim ingested the material several hours before symptoms of toxicity occurred, it is wasting valuable time to try and induce vomiting. Call for professional help IMMEDIATELY.

GENERAL GUIDES:

1) Keep the victim as calm as possible. Panicking and hysteria increase the speed with which the poison invades the system.

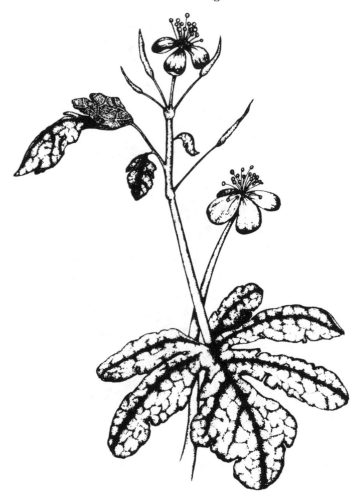

GREATER CELANDINE (*Chelidonium majus*) is a vociferous poison. All parts of the plant are dangerous, but especially the rootstock.

2) If you have it available, Ipecac syrup may be given to the victim. 15 ml (½ fl oz) for a child and 45 ml (1½ fl oz) for an adult. This is not a folk remedy for poisoning. Ipecac syrup is recognized as an excellent first-aid treatment for poisoning by orthodox physicians.

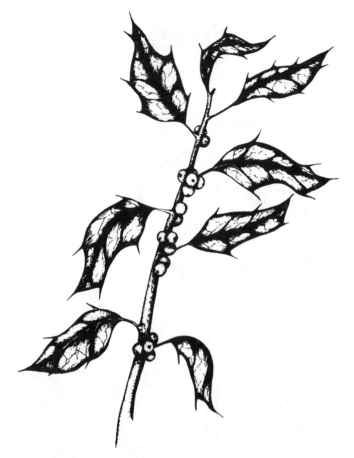

HOLLY (*Ilex aquifolium*) can be used to treat rheumatism, but the berries are extremely poisonous.

3) NEVER clean up or remove vomited material until AFTER your doctor has seen it. Undigested plant material in the vomit can give important clues as to the nature of the toxic material swallowed.

4) Never assume that because vomiting has been induced or the symptoms seem to be lessening in severity that 'the worst is over.' ALL poisoning victims need professional help.

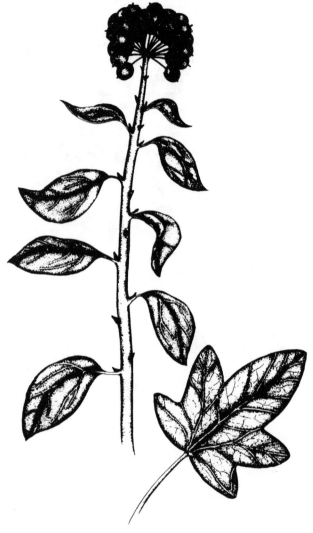

IVY: The various species must be treated with extreme caution as some are
violent poisons.

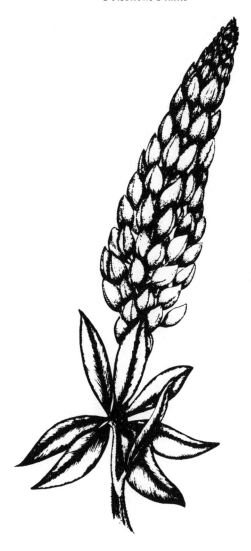

LUPINS (various species) are beautiful in the garden but extremely poisonous.

A TYPICAL POISONS LIST

HERB	COMMON NAME	POISONOUS PART
Aconitum napellus	Monkshood (Aconite)	All, but esp. root
Atropa belladonna	Deadly Nightshade	All
Brassica napus	False Mustard	All
Bryonia dioica	White Bryony	Roots and berries
Caltha palustris	Marsh Marigold	The sap
Chelidonium majus	Greater Celandine	All, but esp. root
Cicuta virosa	Cowbane	Roots, leaves, flowers
Clematis vitalba	Traveller's Joy	All
Conium maculatum	Hemlock	All
Convallaria majalis	Lily Of The Valley	All
Delphinium ajacis	Larkspur	Seeds and leaves
Digitalis purpurea	Foxglove	All
Equisetum arvense	Horsetail	All
Hedera helix	Ivy	Leaves and berries
Helleborus foetida	Stinking Hellebore	All
Ilex aquifolium	Holly	Berries
Laburnum anagyroides	Laburnum	All, esp. bark and seeds
Lupinus (various)	Lupin	All, esp. seeds
Oxalis acetosella	Wood Sorrel	Leaves
Ranunculis acris	Buttercup	The sap
Sarothamnus scoparius	Broom	Seeds
Taxus baccata	Yew	Leaves and seeds
Viscum album	Mistletoe	Berries

Part Three

1 Herbal Medicine Throughout the World's Cultures

If there is one aspect of medical practice that has united the physicians of the world throughout the millenia despite all their diverse opinions, it is their reliance on our flora as a staple source of medicinal drugs.

Virtually all early civilizations developed the use of plant drugs to a high degree. Mineral based drugs were a relatively new development, and had met with a lukewarm response by the medical authorities in many areas, particularly the Americas and central Europe. Each ancient culture seems to have excelled in one particular branch of the tree of medical science; but they *all* made use of plant medicines.

The greatest figure in Egyptian medicine was undoubtedly Imhotep, whose name means 'provider of inner contentment'. He combined his considerable knowledge of the medical sciences with the dignity and compassion of a true healer, and was eventually deified by his fellow countrymen after his death – a move Imhotep himself would undoubtedly have frowned upon.

The Egyptian physicians operated within a professional structure not unlike that of modern orthodox medicine. Experienced practitioners were allowed to become 'specialists' and concentrate their skills on one particular region of the body. Papyrii dealing with medical matters have been unearthed in which mention is made of stomach doctors, upper respiratory tract doctors, eye doctors and so on.

The basic pharmacopoea of the Egyptian physician consisted of around nine hundred herbs, many of them still used today for the same purposes.

As well as possessing considerable expertise in herbology, Egyptian physicians were also skilled in dentistry and dental

Egyptian Pharmacopoeal Herbs	*Traditional Uses*
THORN APPLE	Diseases of the respiratory tract.
POPPY	Sedative and anodyne.
SQUILL	Used as an emetic in cases of poisoning, and as a febrifuge.
HEMLOCK	Diseases of the muscular and nervous system.
MANDRAKE	Liver disorders and impotency.
GENTIAN	As an antibiotic, and as a tonic in cases of general malaise.
CASTOR OIL	Constipation.
SENNA	Constipation, poor digestion and anorexia.
CINNAMON	Stomach disorders.

prosthetics. Embalmed bodies have been unearthed in which dentures have been found wired to the remaining natural teeth. This high level of dental technology was lost when Egyptian civilization declined, and was not regained until the 19th century with the advent of modern European dental skills.

The ancient Indian physicians of the Vedic era excelled in matters of hygiene. They possessed a knowledge of disease prevention and quarantine equalled only by that of the ancient Hebrews. Their true forté however, was in the field of surgery. In some respects the Vedic surgeons had a success rate comparable with that of their modern-day counterparts.

Their unparalleled ingenuity is best highlighted by their method of closing wounds after carrying out internal surgery. The 'old' method of stitching was abandoned and supplanted by the following extraordinary method.

After surgery on the intestines, several large ants were held near the aperture or wound, the edges of which were being held together by an assistant. The ants were irritated by the surgeon and encouraged to bite, and at the very moment when the pincers closed over both sides of the wound the body of the ant was severed from the head. The pincers remained in a locked position and kept the wound closed, whilst the formic acid acted as a sterilizing agent.

In 1953, surgeon Benzo Percival cut open the intestine of several laboratory rats and sealed them again using the ant method. All the rats made a speedy recovery and showed no ill effects.

The ancient Indians were just as ingenious in their used of herbal medicines. Astringent and styptic herbs were used during minor surgical operations to control bleeding, and antiseptic herbal dusting powders were brushed over wounds to reduce the possibility of infection. Surprisingly, the Indian pharmacopoea was smaller than those of several other surrounding nations. Despite their high level of medical sophistication, they saw the wisdom in not complicating matters unnecessarily, and therefore kept a pharmacopoea of just five hundred herbs. There is evidence that a further six or seven hundred plants were used for medicinal purposes on special occasions, but the Vedic surgeons preferred to use a relatively small number of herbs proficiently rather than dabble with others of which their knowledge was lacking.

Indian Pharmacopoeal Herbs	Traditional Uses
RAUWOLFIA	Used to treat hypertension.
QUINCE	Used to treat dysentry and diarrhoea, and as a styptic.
PSYLLIUM	Intestinal inflammation.
ADRUE	Used to treat dyspepsia.
SWEET ALMOND	Used as a laxative.
CATSFOOT	Used as an astringent and antiseptic mouthwash.
FENUGREEK	Stomach ulcers and skin ailments.
ASAFOETIDA	Stomach ailments, rheumatism and various other complaints.

Another ancient civilization that excelled in the medical arts was that of Mesopotamia. Like the ancient Indians, Mesopotamian physicians possessed a high degree of surgical skill, but their pharmocopoea contained a far greater number of herbs. Around fourteen hundred plants were used regularly, although the individual physician or chemist was unlikely to stock anywhere near this amou... on a permanent basis.

In matters pertaining to surgery, Mesopotamian doctors made very few mistakes. They couldn't really afford to, because the surgeon found guilty of negligence was liable to have his hands chopped off as a punishment. This may sound a little barbaric, but I'm sure it did wonders for their powers of concentration.

Mesopotamian physicians imported many of the herbs used for medicinal purposes, and clay tablets detailing their purchase have been unearthed.

Mesopotamian Pharmaco-poeal Herbs	*Traditional Uses*
BELLADONNA	Used to treat epilepsy and nervous spasms.
ASAFOETIDA	Used in cases of rheumatism and as an expectorant.
POPPY	As an anaesthetic.
HENBANE	Used to treat muscular wasting.
LETTUCE	Used as a sedative.
LICORICE	Used to treat respiratory diseases and bowel infections.
PERIWINKLE	Menstrual disorders.
EUPHORBIUM	Used as a purgative in cases of chronic bowel stoppage.
FENNEL	Used as a carminative.
FIG	Used as an antiseptic and natural antibiotic to treat boils and suppurations.

One of the nations with whom the Mesopotamians traded was China. There is evidence that certain herbs – such as *Panax quinquefolia* – were bought by physicians from several Middle-eastern countries from Chinese apothecaries, and as early as 2000 B.C. Chinese physicians even developed a somewhat bizarre, but nonetheless effective, means of innoculating people against the dreaded disease smallpox. The scabs of a dead smallpox victim were removed from the corpse and dried. Then they were comminuted into a fine powder which was blown into the nose of the person to be innoculated.

Like the Mesopotamians, the Chinese had a large pharmacopoea.

Many of the Chinese medicinal herbs were recognized as efficacious only by Chinese physicians.

Chinese Pharmacopoeal Herbs	Traditional Uses
GINSENG	Used as a tonic and general restorative. Also given to enhance the action of other herbs.
CHESTNUT	Used to treat respiratory illnesses.
NUTMEG	Heart disease.
POMEGRANATE	Used as a vermifuge.
EPHEDRA	Used to treat asthma and related conditions.
SHENZI RHUBARB	Used as an aperient.
CANTONESE RHUBARB	Used in small doses to cure diarrhoea, and conversely, in larger doses as a laxative.

Of all the medico-cultures of the early civilizations, the ancient Israelites were in some respects unique. The medical philosophies of virtually all the other nations were steeped in demonology, magic and astrology, whereas the Hebrews, except for one or two turbulent periods in their history, remained free from such influence. they had no time for spells, incantations and magic formulas and only borrowed those medical concepts from the surrounding nations that were proveable either by cold logic or physical demonstration.

The Hebrews were not as scrupulous in the keeping of secular records as they were with their ecclesiastical ones, and so a great deal of valuable information concerning ancient Jewish medicine has been lost. But much remains, and that which we possess demonstrates most clearly that they possessed a staggering degree of medical ability.

The hygiene laws of Israel were second to none. One has only to read Dr. Roswell Park's book *An Epitome Of The History of Medicine* to see the ghastly effects of the lack of hygiene in British hospitals in the 19th century, but as S. I. McMillen comments in *None Of These Diseases* (Fleming H. Revell, 1963),

Such mortality would not have occurred if surgeons had only followed the method God gave to Moses regarding the meticulous method of hand washing and changing of clothes after contact with infectious diseases.

The Hebrew pharmacopoea was not as vast as that of the Chinese or Mesopotamians, but as mineral based drugs were out of favour with Jewish physicians, the herbs that they did use were employed frequently and had their effects well documented.

Hebrew Pharmacopoeal Herbs	*Traditional Uses*
CINNAMON	Used in the treatment of stomach ailments.
FIG	Antiseptic and antibiotic.
BALM	Used as an emolient and for certain skin ailments.
ORANGE	Used to treat respiratory ailments and certain skin diseases.
MANDRAKE	Not exactly known, possibly in the treatment of impotence and dropsy.
GINSENG	Not exactly known, but the herb is alluded to in the Bible and seems to have been highly valued.

But to suggest that the Middle and Far East were the only areas that developed botanic medicine to a high degree would be misleading. Another centre of intense herbal activity was the Americas. The Amerindians have a long and fascinating history of 'green medicine', and Amerindian herbology is a detailed subject in itself. The main contribution of the American Indians towards the practice of herbalism lies in the fact that they were the first to develop the Doctrine Of Signatures, and at this juncture it would be prudent to digress for a moment and discuss just what the Doctrine Of Signatures is.

Ancient Indian medicine men guarded their knowledge jealously. The art of healing was viewed, quite correctly, as a noble one, the secrets of which were not to be divulged to just anyone who happened to enquire of them. And so, no written pharmacopoea was kept. Each medicine man passed down his accumulated wisdom to his apprentice who, in turn guarded it jealously.

But of course, no medicine man could possibly be expected – no matter how learned – to remember every medicinal herb and its properties. The Amerindian pharmacopoea was an oral one, but large nevertheless, and the medicine men knew that when a large body of information was passed orally error could easily creep in.

To counteract the possibility of mistakes being made, a fascinating mnemonic system was developed which enabled the user to remember the medicinal qualities of an individual plant. It is this system that is generally called the Doctrine Of Signatures.

Quite simply, it works like this. A medicine man would study the external appearance of a plant and find something about it that would help the user remember what it should be used for. Noon Flower (*Tragopogon pratens*) was a popular remedy for jaundice. The healer was reminded of this by the vivid yellow colour of the flower heads. Lesser Scabious (*Scabiosa columbaria*) was used in the treatment of skin ailments. The signature' of the plant was the scaly pappus found on the seeds. This looked like the scaling diseases of the skin that the herb could be used to treat.

Commonly Used Amerindian Herbs	*Traditional Uses*
JUNIPER BERRY	Used to treat kidney ailments.
CULVER'S ROOT	Used as a laxative.
LYCOPODIUM	Antiseptic and styptic (used in powder form).
HOREHOUND	Diseases of the respiratory tract.
BLOODROOT	Gastric stimulant and expectorant.
AMERICAN BLACK HAW	Used to treat dysmenorrhoea.
SLIPPERY ELM	Intestinal disorders.

Herbal Faculties and Colleges

Choosing a competent Herbalist is a bit like walking through a therapeutic minefield. When I inform my orthodox colleagues that there are actually over two hundred faculties and colleges in the British Isles teaching herbalism and other unorthodox therapies, their reaction is normally one of extreme scepticism. In truth, the average person in the street is usually unaware that there is *any* formal method of training for a career in herbal medicine, but the current boom in interest has seen a plethora of small 'colleges' spring up alongside the handful of more established ones.

It is vitally important that those who wish to consult a herbal practitioner are able to determine the value of his or her qualifications. Whilst there are many excellent herbalists in practice who have no formal qualifications whatsoever, there are a number who have little or no experience but who hide behind a bogus list of qualifications that mean absolutely nothing.

Some 'colleges' are little more than degree mills that will supply an impressive looking certificate in return for a £10 cheque or Postal Order, no questions asked. On the other hand, the respectable faculties usually make their students go through years of arduous training, ensuring that they are fully competent before they unleash their talents on the general public. The majority, however, fall between these two polarities.

ACUPUNCTURE AND CHINESE HERBAL PRACTITION-ERS TRAINING COLLEGE.

199a, Gloucester Place, London, NW1 6BU.

The most impressive of those faculties which specialize in the more traditional forms of Oriental medicine.

Besides teaching acupuncture, the college also runs intensive weekend and evening courses in herbal medicine. All the presiding tutors are Chinese and are genuinely qualified.

Their prospectus is well prepared and bears none of the usual hallmarks of quackery.

Although their training course involves a little less practical instruction than the courses run by some other faculties, it seems that students are expected to reach a high standard. Thoroughly recommended.

COLLEGE OF NATURAL THERAPY,
4, Overbury Road, Lower Parkstone, Poole, Dorset.

Before taking their diploma course in Herbal Medicine, all students are required to take an introductory course in anatomy and physiology. This includes fourteen detailed studies of the human body beginning with 'Cells – The Basis For Life'. The course also covers the Circulatory System (two parts), Digestion, Reproduction and all other body systems.

The course in herbalism is comprehensive and erudite, and contains a seven-part *Materia Medica*. It emphasizes the theoretical basis of modern herbalism most strongly, and all students are furnished with a poisons schedule that lists those herbs unsuitable for use because of their toxic effects.

Practical training is given.

THE FACULTY OF HERBAL MEDICINE,
'Merlynne', Meadfoot Close, Ilsham Road, Torquay, TQ1 2JJ, South Devon.

The teaching arm of the The General Council And Register Of Consultant Herbalists.

This is one of the oldest teaching faculties in the U.K. and is itself a splinter group of the National Institute of Medical Herbalists. The faculty has an excellent teaching programme that is, in the author's opinion, superior in some ways to that of the NIMH, although the training does not seem quite so intensive.

The college also makes the study of anatomy and physiology compulsory for students.

Many faculty members can be numbered amongst the U.K.'s most accomplished practitioners.

GALEN COLLEGE, 78–79, Pinfold Street, Darlaston, Wednesbury, West Midlands, WS10 8TB

Offers a correspondence course in Herbology (an Americanism for Herbal Medicine) and awards a certificate at the end of it.

Ideal for those who want a general grounding in Herbalism without becoming involved in practical training.

THE INSTITUTE OF ALTERNATIVE MEDICINE,
310, Kennington Road, London, SW11.

Offers part time evening and weekend courses in Herbal Medicine with practical seminars. Seems to be well organized.

MODERN ACADEMY OF INTERNATIONAL HERBAL MEDICINE,
40, Crown Dale, London, SE19

Offers a two year correspondence course in Herbal Medicine.

THE NATIONAL INSTITUTE OF MEDICAL HEBALISTS.
41, Hatherley Road, Winchester, Hampshire. S022 6RR.

The NIMH is the oldest and largest of those institutes that teach herbalism as a profession. It runs a four year course that gives students a thorough grounding in all the medical sciences, and includes a high degree of practical training.

Many graduates of the Institute have written books on Herbal Medicine, and this body more than any other has been responsible for giving the craft its current air of respectability and sober professionalism. The NIMH has done much to try and foster good relations between British herbalists and the orthodox profession, although the response has often been lukewarm to say the least.

BRANTRIDGE FOREST SCHOOL,
Highfield, Dane Hill, Haywards Heath, Sussex, RH17 7EX.

Offers a wide variety of courses in many 'alternative' medical subjects, including Botanic Medicine or Herbalism. The course is geared to the individual student, reasonably priced and includes a range of superb text books.

Most of the course material is written by one of England's most prolific writers on the subject, Professor Donald Law, and supplemented by material from the Dean of the School, Professor Bruce Copen.

Most of the material cannot be found in other courses or text books on the subject, and although the student will undoubtedly find some of the School's ideas radical and controversial, it gives excellent instruction on botany, the ecology and similar subjects.

CORRESPONDENCE COURSES IN CANADA AND THE U.S.A.

DOMINION HERBAL COLLEGE,
7527, Kingsway, Burnaby, British Columbia, V3N 3C1, Canada.

Canada's most distinguished herbal college; first instituted in 1926 and respected worldwide.

The college gives detailed training in anatomy and physiology, and also covers dietetics as well as the main section on herbalism. Other subjects are dealt with that are not covered by other faculties in any detail, such as veterinary herbalism.

Perhaps the college's most powerful reference is its distinguished list of students. These include the author and nutritionist Dr. Edward Fewer, and the iridologist Dr. Bernard Jensen.

SCHOOL OF NATURAL HEALING, Box 352, Provo, Utah, 84601, U.S.A.

One of America's best herbal colleges. This course provides an exhaustive foundation in all aspects of Herbology, is scientifically correct and does not give in to the 'cash in on the great herbal bonanza now' approach of other 'colleges'.

The course is run by Ray Christopher, a leading U.S. herbal expert.

THE INSTITUTE OF HERBAL PHILOSOPHY,
Box 968, 115 East Foothill No. 10, Glendora, California, 91740.

The Institute is (was?) run by schoolteacher/herbalist Gene Matlock. It emphasises the practise of herbalism by ancient civilizations such as the Aztecs and Chinese, and also provides instruction on how to make a financial success out of the various aspects of the profession.

I recently wrote to the Institute asking for a current prospectus, but my letter was returned with the legend 'moved on – no forwarding address' written on it.

A Guide to Herbal Literature

There is a large library of books on Herbalism available, much of it good, a lot of it mediocre and some just downright deplorable. What I offer here is just a smattering, but even the bad ones are worth reading if for nothing more than their entertainment value.

Green Pharmacy Barbara Griggs.
   The best introduction to the history of herbal medicine available. The various chapters analyse the development of herbalism through the ages, and nearly all of the profession's noteable characters are biographed. Not to be missed. Published by Jill Norman & Hobhouse Ltd.

Alternative Medicine Robert Eagle.
   A fascinating excursion into the more bizarre caverns of alternative medicine, with a comprehensive chapter on herbalism.
   The author tends to be overly cynical when dealing with some of the more controversial aspects of alternative medicine in general, but his book provides a goldmine of historical nuggets which gives those interested in herbal medicine an intriguing insight into the minds of some of its intellectual giants. Published by Futura Publications.

Some Good Herbs Alfred K. Barrals. (U.S.A.)
   A tatty book containing totally erroneous information about fifty medicinal herbs.
   I have tried to trace both the author and the publisher (without success) to see how they managed to get away publishing such a potentially dangerous piece of rubbish which recommends swallowing small quantities of Deadly Nightshade for colic. Both the publisher and the writer have disappeared from the scene – probably to South America to escape the wrath of America's Herbalists proper. Published by Berpilip Now – whoever they are.

Herbs for Headaches and Migraine Nalda Gosling.

One of the popular 'Everybody's Home Herbal' series that can be found in many health food stores and direct from the publishers.

An interesting guide to how various herbs such as Couchgrass, Lime and Motherwort can be used to relieve headaches. Others in the series deal with the skin, kidneys, eyes, digestion etc., Published by Thorsons.

The Herbal or General Historie of Plantes John Gerard.

Gerard can rightfully be regarded as England's first master herbalist. Unlike his contemporaries, he was not given to fanciful old wives' tales based on superstition and myth. In the main, his findings are based on factual observances during his years of experience.

The book was first published in 1597 and is still occasionally reprinted. Gerard has a mischievous sense of humour that makes the book extremely entertaining, as well as giving a fascinating glimpse at the practice of mediaeval medicine. Various publishers.

Potter's New Cyclopaedia of Botanical Drugs and Preparations R. C. Wren.

If you're really serious about herbal medicine then you should make strenuous efforts to get this book. Hundreds of herbs are listed A–Z style, and each heading gives information concerning the habitat of the plant, flowering times and, most importantly, notes on dosage.

One of the few herbals that doesn't leave you irritated because important detials have been left out. Published by The C. W. Daniel Co. Ltd.

Modern Encyclopedia of Herbs Joseph M. Kadans.

A handy A–Z of herbs that provides a lot of information about some of the more obscure herbs – some of them quite rare – that grow in the U.S.A. Besides discussing the more popular plant remedies, Kadans also includes others such as Pukeweed and Squaw-root.

Kadans has cut through a lot of the dross and produced a book that gives all the essential details without leaving the reader bored stiff. Also includes a 'Herb-O-Matic locator index' which enables the herbs to be cross-referenced with various diseases. Published by

Parker Publishing Co, New York, and Thorsons Publishers (re-titled 'Encyclopedia Of Medicinal Herbs'), England.

The Compleat Herbal Ben Charles Harris.

Written by one of the brightest stars in the American herbal firmament. This book is different. The author has spent much time researching the herbal lore of the American indians, and this gives a distinctive 'back to nature' feel to it. If you want a book that captures that spirit of American pioneer herbalism, but which is factually accurate at the same time, then this is it. Don't miss it. Published by Larchmont.

Culpeper's Herbal Nicholas Culpeper.

Culpeper is synonymous with English herbalism, and there is a distinct idea amongst many who follow him that every word that dripped from the nib of his quill should be treated as Holy Writ.

In fact, although Culpeper's work is a valuable work in many ways, it leaves a lot to be desired. Unlike his predecessor John Gerard, Culpeper allowed his intellectual brilliance to be tainted by his deep belief in astrology. Thus, it is difficult to determine which of his conclusions are based on his medical experience as opposed to those which are the result of his star-gazing.

Most herbalists have a copy of 'Culpeper' not because it is a superlative piece of herbal literature, but simply because it's the 'done thing'. Various publishers.

Herbal Suppliers

A quick perusal of some of the sundry health magazines available in health food stores and newsagents will yield a host of suppliers who market dried herbs. The following are reputable companies who supply high quality products.

Down to Earth,
3, The Grove,
Coulsdon,
Surrey,
CR3 2BH.

Cross House Cottage,
Layer de la Have,
Nr. Colchester,
Essex.

Rayner & Pennycook,
No. 6, Rayvit House,
Shepperton,
Middlesex.

Midland Herbs & Spices,
5a, Formans Trading Estate,
Pentos Drive,
Sparkhill,
Birmingham,
B11 3TA.

Cornucopia Wholefoods,

64, St. Mary's Road,
Ealing,
London,
W5 5EX.

G. Baldwin & Co,
173, Walworth Road,
London,
SE17 1RW.
(This company stock the widest range of herbal products I've ever seen.)

Black Forest House Of Herbs,
32, Forestdale,
London,
N14 7DX.
(This company airmail in speciality German herbal teas for the customer from Europe. They are on the expensive side (just), but don't let that put you off. The extra quality makes up for the 2 or 3 pence they add on to the price of an ounce.)

There are many herb suppliers in the U.S.A., and the best way to keep tabs on them is to read THE HERB QUARTERLY (West Street, New Fane, Vermont, 05345, USA) which carries advertisements from reputable suppliers.

Appendices

Appendix A   Dosage Tables

The following chart is a general guide to determining the percentage of 1 complete dose that should be given to patients of various ages. However, other factors must be considered. These include the weight, sex and general health of the patient. The controlling dose is one adult measure.

Age of Patient	Fraction of One Whole Dose Required
1 mo.	1/12 to 1/10 (taken under direction)
2–12 mo.	1/12 to 1/10
1–2 yrs.	1/10 to 1/8
2–3 yrs.	1/8 to 1/6
3–4 yrs.	1/6
4–5 yrs.	1/6 to 1/4
5–6 yrs.	1/4
6–8 yrs.	1/4 to 1/3
8–10 yrs.	1/3
10–12 yrs.	1/3 to 1/2
12–14 yrs.	1/2 to 2/3
14–18 yrs.	2/3 to 3/4
18/40 yrs.	1
40–60 yrs.	7/8
60–80 yrs.	2/3 to 3/4
80 +	1/2 to 2/3

Appendix B Weights and Measures Tables

Avoirdupois.

16 drams	=	1 oz.	(437.5 grains)
16 oz.	=	1 lb.	(7,000 grains.)
14 lbs.	=	1 Stone.	
28 lbs.	=	1 quarter.	
4 quarters	=	1 hundredweight.(112 lbs.)	
20 hundredweight	=	1 Ton.	(2,240 lbs.)

Metric.

10 milligrams	=	1 centigram.	(0.154 grains)
10 centigrams	=	1 decigram.	(1.543 grains)
10 decigrams	=	1 gram.	(15.432 grains)
10 grams	=	1 decagram	(0.3527 avoirdupois ounces.)
10 decagrams	=	1 hectogram	(3.5274 avoirdupois ounces.)
10 hectograms	=	1 kilogram	(2.2046 pounds.)

Metric (Volume).

10 centimils	=	1 decimil	(1.6894 minims.)
10 decimils	=	1 mil (c.c.)	(16.8941 minims.)
10 mils	=	1 centilitre	(2.8157 fluid drachms)
100 mils	=	1 decilitre	(3.5196 fluid ounces)
1,000 mils	=	1 litre	(1.7598 pints)

Apothecary weight.

20 grains	=	1 scruple.
3 scruples	=	1 drachm.
8 drachms	=	1 ounce.

Apothecary Fluid Measure.

60 minims	=	1 fluid drachm.
8 fluid drachms	=	1 fluid ounce.
20 fluid ounces	=	1 pint.
2 pints	=	1 quart.
4 quarts	=	1 gallon.

Appendix C   Common Medical Abbreviations

aa.	ana	of each
a.c.	ante cibum	before food
ad lib.	ad libitum	as much as required
alt. die.	alternis diebus	alternate days
ante jentac.	ante jentaculum	to be taken before breakfast
aq.	aqua	in water
b.i.d.	bis in die	twice a day
c.	cum	with
cat.	cataplasma	a poultice
coch.	cochleare	a spoonful
cochl. mag.	cochleare magnum	a tablespoonful
cochl. min.	cocheare minimum	a teaspoonful
conc.	concentratus	concentrated
dil.	dilue	diluted
ext.	extractum	extraction
garg.	gargarisma	a gargle
in.d.	in dies	in a day, daily
inf.	infusum	an infusion
inj.	injectio	by injection
lin.	linimentum	liniment
liq.	liquor	in solution
mist.	mistura	a mixture
par.aeq.	partes aequales	in equal amounts
p.c.	post cibum	after food
p.r.	per rectum	by the rectum
q.s.	quantum sufficit	in sufficient amounts
t.d.s.	ter in die sumendus	three times a day

Appendix D Orthodox and Unorthodox Medical Letters, Degrees and Diplomas

A.B.	Bachelor of Arts
A.B.I.H.	Member Associate of The British Institute of Health
A.D.M.S.	Assistant Director of Medical Services
A.H.H.S.A.	American Holistic Health Sciences Association
A.H.P.	Assistant House Physician
A.H.S.	Assistant House Surgeon
A.R.San.I.	Associate of the Royal Sanitary Institute
B.A.	Bachelor of Arts
B.A.O.	Bachelor of Obstetrics
B.C.	Bachelor of Surgery
B.Ch.	Bachelor of Surgery
B.Ch.D.	Bachelor of Dental Surgery
B.D.S.	Bachelor of Dental Surgery
B.H.H.S.A.	British Holistic Health Sciences Association
B.Hy.	Bachelor of Hygiene
B.M.	Bachelor of Medicine
B.M.A.	British Medical Association
B.S.	Bachelor of Surgery
B.Sc.	Bachelor of Science
D.A.	Diploma in Anaesthetics
D.Ac.	Diploma in Acupuncture
D.Ac.	Doctor of Acupuncture
D.Bio.	Diploma in Schuessler's Biochemistry
D.B.M.	Diploma in Botanic Medicine
D.Ch.O.	Diploma in Opthalmic Surgery
D.Chrom.	Diploma in Chromotherapy
Lic. Ac.	Licentiate in Acupuncture
L.M.S.	Licentiate in Medical Surgery
M.A.O.	Master of Obstetrics
M.B.H.U.	Member of The British Herbalists' Union
M.B.I.H.	Member of The British Institute of Health
M.B.N.O.A.	Member of The British Naturopathic and Osteopathic Association

M.C.N.T.	Member of The College of Natural Therapy
M.C.O.	Member of The College of Osteopaths
M.D.S.	Master of Dental Surgery
M.H.	Master of Hygiene
M.L.C.O.M.	Member of The London College of Osteopathic Medicine
M.R.H.	Member of The Register of Herbalists
M.R.O.	Member of The Register of Osteopaths
M.S.	Master of Science (Nutrition)
N.D.	Doctor of Naturopathy
N.D.	Diploma in Naturopathy
N.D.	Diploma in Natural Sciences
Ph.D.	Doctor of Philosophy
P.M.O.	Principal Medical Officer
R.H.P.	Registered Homoeopathic Practitioner
R.M.H.	Registered Medical Herbalist
R.N.	Registered Nurse
R.O.	Registered Osteopath
S.C.M.	State Certified Midwife
S.R.N.	State Registered Nurse
D.Dt	Diploma in Dietetics
D.D.H.	Diploma in Drugless Healing
D.G.O.	Diploma in Gynaecology and Obstetrics
D. Hom.	Diploma in Homoeopathy
D.Hom.	Doctor of Homoeopathy
D.Ho.M.	Diploma in Homoeopathic Medicine
D.H.Med.	Diploma in Herbal Medicine
D.Hy.	Diploma in Hygiene
D.Hy.	Doctor of Hygiene
D.M.	Doctor of Medicine
D.M.R.	Diploma in Medical Radiology
D.N.	Diploma in Nursing
D.O.	Diploma in Osteopathy
D.O.	Doctorate in Osteopathy
D.P.M.	Diploma in Psychological Medicine
D.Phil.	Dctor of Philosophy
D.Psy.	Diploma in Psychology
D.Psych.	Diploma in Psychotherapy
D.Sc.	Doctor of Science
F.A.C.P.	Fellow of The American College of Physicians
F.B.I.H.	Fellow of The British Institute of Health
F.C.O.	Fellow of the College of Osteopaths
F.H.M.	Faculty of Herbal Medicine
F.L.C.O.M.	Fellow of The London College of Osteopathic Medicine

F.R.I.P.H.	Fellow of The Royal Institute of Public Health
H.P.A.	Health Prctitioners' Association
I.A.N.C.	International Academy of Nutritional Consultants
I.C.A.N.	International College of Applied Nutrition

Index

INDEX

ABOUT THE AUTHOR

Michael Hallowell first began his career in medicine when he studied dental prosthetics at Newcastle University Dental Hospital, but quickly became intrigued by unorthodox therapies during discussions with a colleague who had studied herbal medicine in China.

After several years researching the subject he gained a Diploma in Botanic Medicine and began a successful occasional practice.

In 1980 he began to lecture widely on the subject and now runs several newspaper and magazine columns on herbal medicine and related subjects. He also contributes to several health journals in the U.S.A.

Besides pursuing his writing career and running a busy practice, Michael Hallowell also takes part in radio and T.V. debates on a variety of medical topics.